The Flat Tummy Book

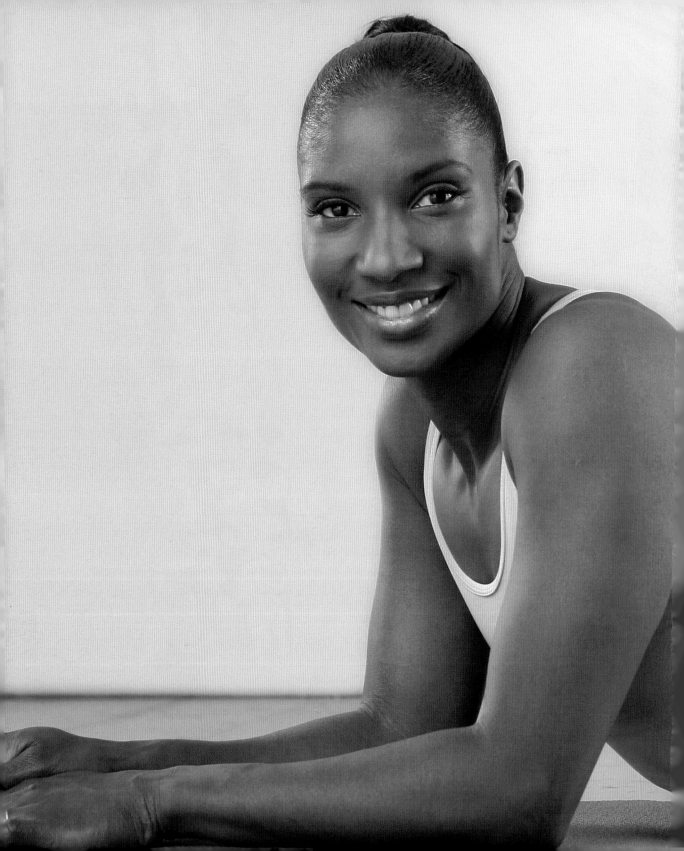

Denise Lewis

The Flat Tummy Book

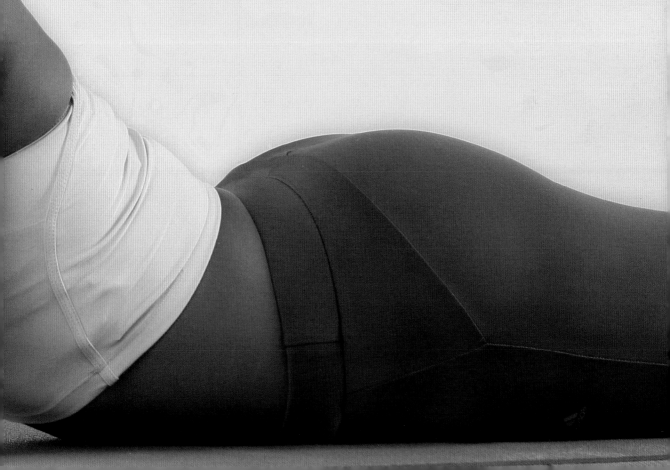

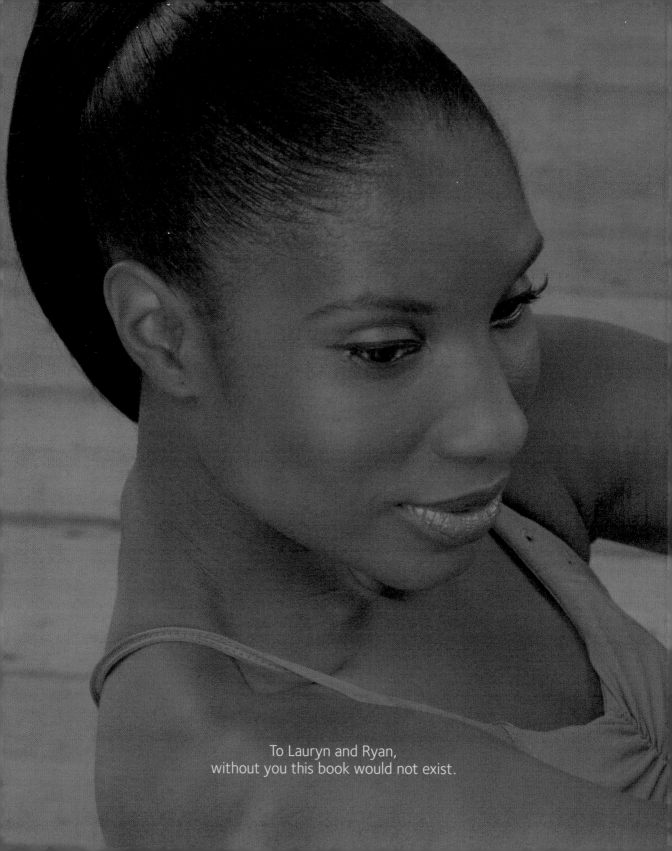

To Lauryn and Ryan,
without you this book would not exist.

Contents

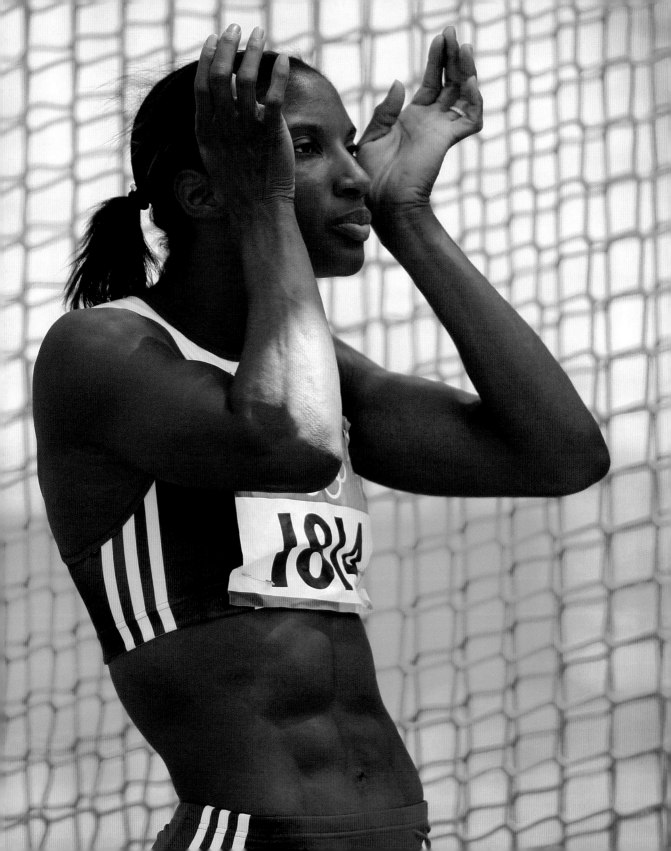

Introduction

I was lucky enough to discover the joys of being active at an early age. I enjoyed the sense of feeling alive whenever I could run around, play ball games or put on my ballet shoes to go dancing; I think I was a normal sort of child. My desire to be an athlete came at the age of eight when I watched my first Olympics on television. I was hooked. I wanted to be like those amazing athletes, and that was all the motivation I needed to make sport my career.

I've watched my body changing over the years and at times I've not appreciated those changes. During my teens for example the developing muscles in my arms and legs didn't cooperate with my desire to be petite and feminine like the other girls I saw on the dance floor or at the bars I occasionally went to. But I loved athletics and my Olympic ambitions drove me onwards – to be the best in the world I needed my strong shapely legs even if it meant forsaking that gorgeous mini skirt.

It wasn't easy, but every year I learned more about my body – what it was capable of physically and how it responded to the investment I put into it. I discovered that you could make changes if you had faith in your own ability. With enough persistance you will succeed.

Making changes doesn't happen overnight: becoming Olympic champion took me twenty long years of hard training. But I had a goal and each day, each week, each month I could feel myself moving closer to it. Setting a goal and visualising where you want to be in the long term is is a vital part of success in any endeavour.

I am very proud of my achievements and that I managed to compete to the best of my ability to win medals for my country. What could be more physically and mentally challenging than that?

Well how about being a mother!

(Left) Preparing for the high jump, Athens Olympics, 2004.

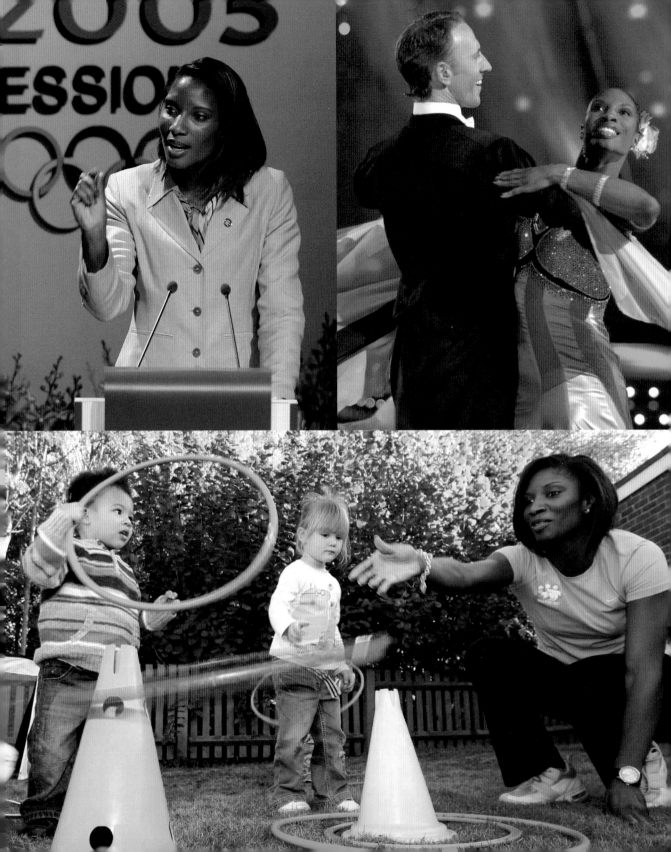

With my first child Lauryn, I had a good pregnancy, ate well, and got back into training. The support of my mum and friends gave me the strength and flexibility to get my Denise Lewis 'the athlete' hat back on.

After a succession of injuries I decided it was time to hang up my spikes and enter a new phase of family life. A year later I gave birth to Ryan my beautiful baby boy weighing a whopping 9lbs. Liberated from the obligations of training, there was a period when I felt quite euphoric. I wanted to indulge in everything naughty, eating and drinking what I liked and when I liked with no thought to working out. I had no desire to. With a new baby in tow, how could I possibly find the time? Every day was one big treat after another. It was an existence that I'd not been used to and I was enjoying my new sense of freedom.

Have you noticed how clever weight is? It sneaks up on you. That's what happened to me and I couldn't see it. It was post-pregnancy weight I thought, not a big deal. But when I saw a picture of myself, I was forced to take a look at my naked body in the mirror.

Strange as it might seem, I was suddenly very self-conscious. For half my life people had talked about my 'six-pack' and my 'washboard stomach' – the person looking back at me had neither of these. I would probably never know that chiselled body again as training six hours a day was no longer an option and I would have to accept that fact.

Half my mind was still thinking I should hit the deck and throw in an instant hundred sit-ups, but I resisted and thought sensibly, 'you can manage how you look and feel comfortable with yourself.' I didn't need a washboard stomach, I just want it to be flat.

(Top left) Presenting London's 2012 Olympic bid;
(Top right) On the dancefloor with Ian Waite in Strictly Come Dancing;
(Left) With my son Ryan at the Youth Sport Trust's Early Years Project.

With this new sense of purpose, I set about designing an exercise programme that took into account a working week with two kids, accommodating the school run and the baby's sleeping times plus the other bits of work I had to do, as well as preparing dinner for the family and getting some sleep.

I knew that the freedom to exercise for as long as I liked was no longer an option and I had taken for granted the luxury that being a full time athlete gave me to be fit and healthy. Finding any time was not going to be easy, but it was up to me to make space in my day and to ensure that my workout was as efficient as possible.

I realised that I could only spare two thirty minute sessions a week to get a flat tummy. It might not sound like enough, but I knew what really works and that's consistency and dedication. If you're doing the right exercises and you repeat them often enough you will get a positive change because that's simply how the body operates.

The road to a flat tummy starts here. The exercises in this book are simple. They don't need much space or time. They worked for me, they'll work for you too. You just have to make the commitment to do them.

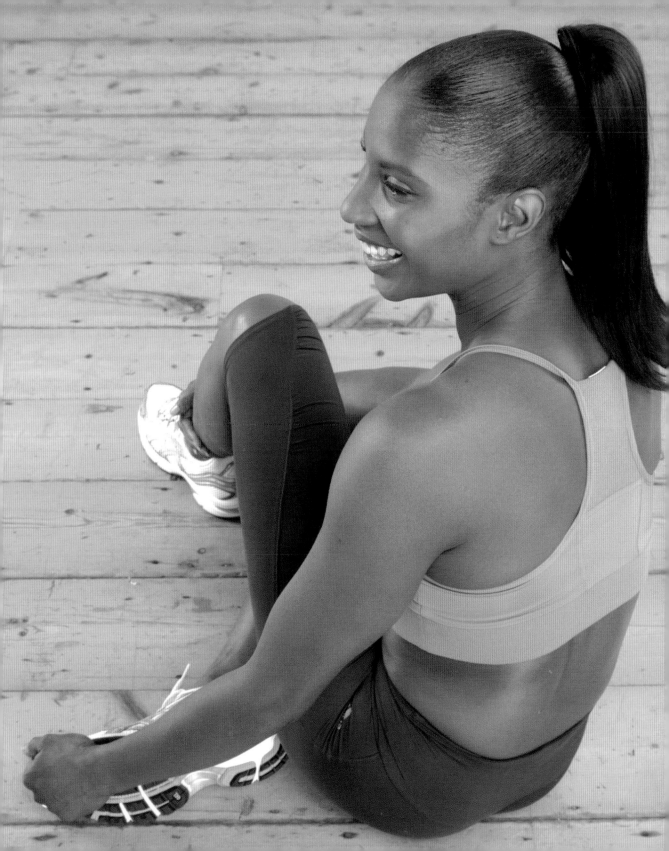

Why Exercise?

'We exercise because we want to look good or feel healthier, and since we should all define our own sense of what looking good is, this book is designed to help you get closer to where you would like to be.'

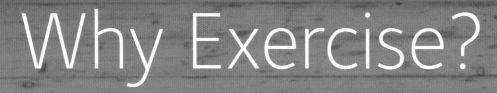

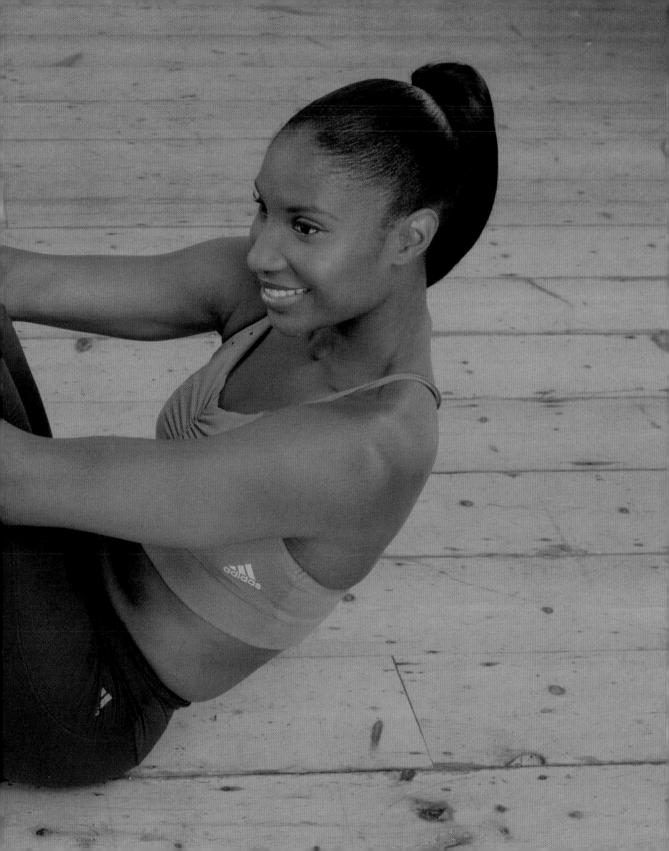

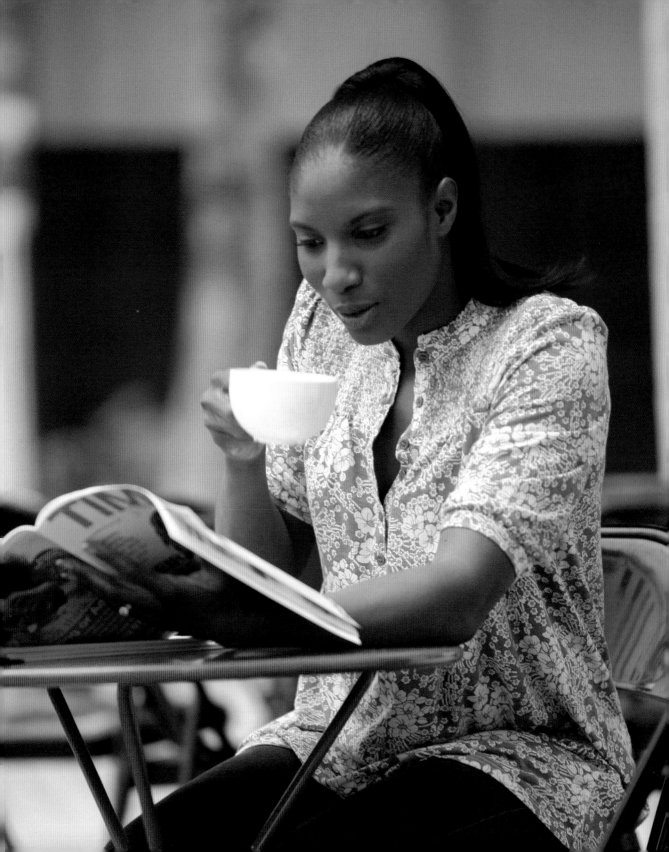

Looking good and feeling good

Let's face it, we tend not to think about the long-term benefits of exercising. We don't think, my heart will be stronger and my lungs will function better. We exercise because we want to look good. We have short-term reasons for getting into shape, perhaps a wedding dress to fit into or a beach holiday we want to look good for.

We should all define our own sense of what looking good is, and this book is designed to help you get closer to where you would like to be.

Believe it or not exercising gives you confidence, because people become more confident from being in better shape than they were and ladies, if you have ever managed to drop a dress size, didn't you feel great!

I know exercise can increase self-esteem. I didn't feel great being at home post pregnancy, even though I was doing one of the most important jobs in the world. But when I re-introduced exercise into my week, my energy levels increased, I coped better with the day's challenges and generally my spirits were up.

Time spent exercising isn't time lost – it's time invested. Finding space in your week to workout will give you an unexpected boost and lead to greater productivity in whatever you are doing – and hopefully you will have a little bit of fun too.

Getting Started

'Having the right attitude will help you stick at it and once you get going you will feel better about yourself and your body.'

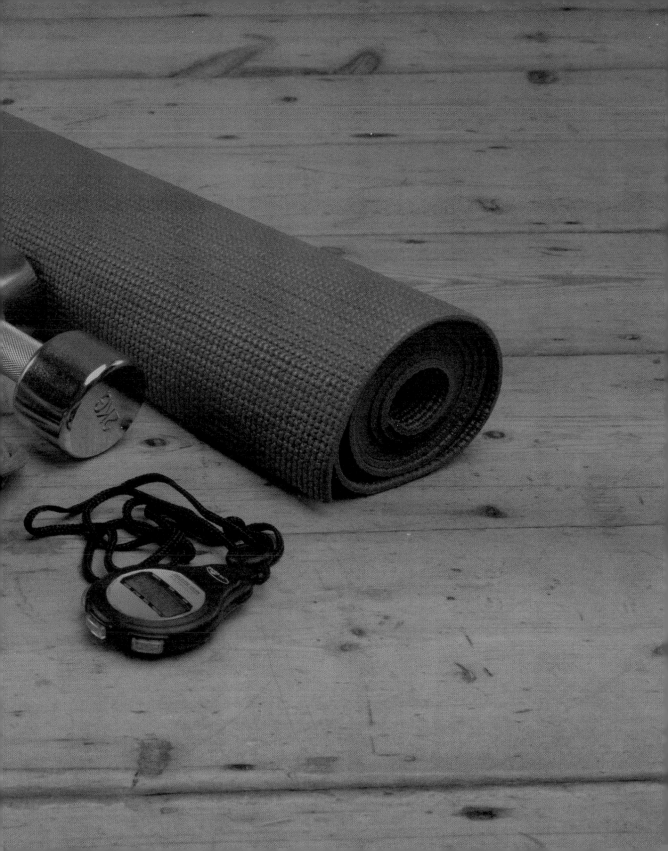

Getting your brain into gear

You probably know as well as I do that maintaining consistent eating habits and exercise is the way to go, but it's not easy with the busy lifestyles we all lead. Managing your time on a day-to-day basis and setting realistic goals is the key to a successful relationship between you and working out.

After having my son Ryan it was extremely difficult to find a routine again. Not only had I lost my athlete's time management skills, I'd also lost time for 'ME'. I had to enlist the help of my husband, who reminded me just how successful I had been getting into shape before. I had the discipline, so I knew I could do it again – but first I had to find a time of day when I would not feel guilty about leaving other tasks until I had given time to 'ME'.

My workout times were either during Ryan's late morning sleep or after bedtime for both children around 7pm. On the days I opted for the evening, I would ask my husband to be home early so he could put them to bed. That way I could exercise, prepare dinner and we were still able to eat together.

Preparing your mental attitude is crucial. Setting a goal – which I am assuming is to get a flat tummy – deciding when you can exercise and reminding yourself to be positive are good starting points. If you decide to work out in the morning, wake up forty minutes earlier to give you time before your day gets going. It is not impossible to do my flat tummy exercises before breakfast, you could have some hot water and honey before you work out just to line the stomach.

If it's more realistic to set time aside in the evening, allow no distractions when you get home. This is probably the hardest time of the day for most people. If you have had a tough day at work, then lying on the sofa may be a more appealing option at this point. Let friends or family help, they can be your allies in motivating you.

Having the right attitude will help you stick at it and once you get going you will feel better about yourself and your body but remember. . . change does not happen overnight.

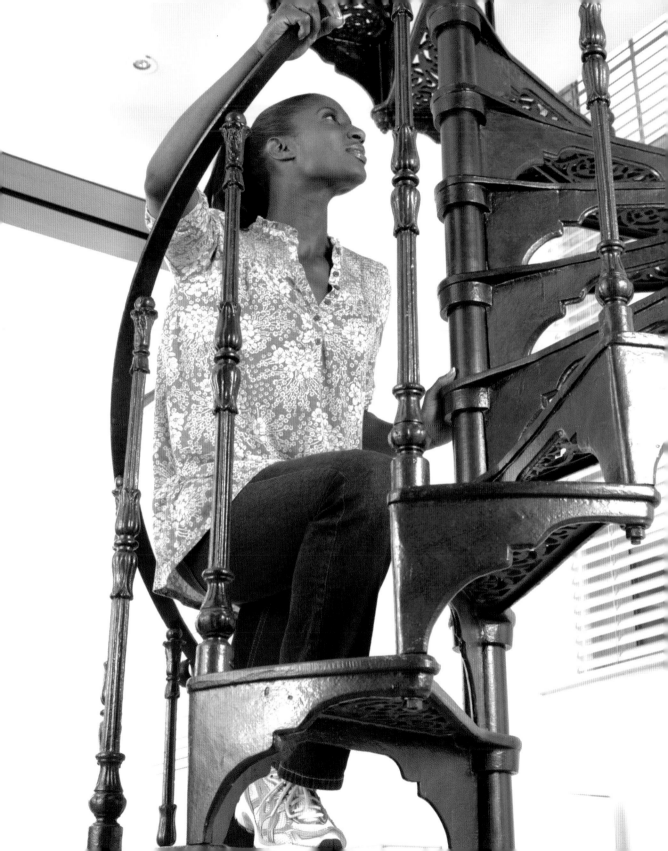

What you need

The point of this book is that you should be able to do these exercises any time, any place and just about anywhere. All you need to do is clear a small space for a dynamic warm up, some easy stretches and then the exercises. Also make sure that there is a flat wall accessible for use. No fancy gadgets or machines are needed, just practical items that you may have at home already or can pick up at the shops cheaply.

All you require is:
* A floor mat
* A good pair of trainers
* A skipping rope for warm up
* Two small cushions and a towel for extra lower back support

* A stopwatch for timed exercises
* A 2 kilo weight
  (You can substitute a 1.5 litre bottle of water or a 2 kilo bag of rice for the 2 kilo weight)

   It is important to wear appropriate clothing for working out, starting off with a comfortable, well supported sports bra or well fitted crop top. Looking after your breasts during any form of exercise is a must!

   The rest of your clothing should be comfortable and unrestrictive, so avoid zips or buttons in tricky places for example.

   Personally, I love to workout listening to music. There's nothing like hearing a good tune to get you in the mood.

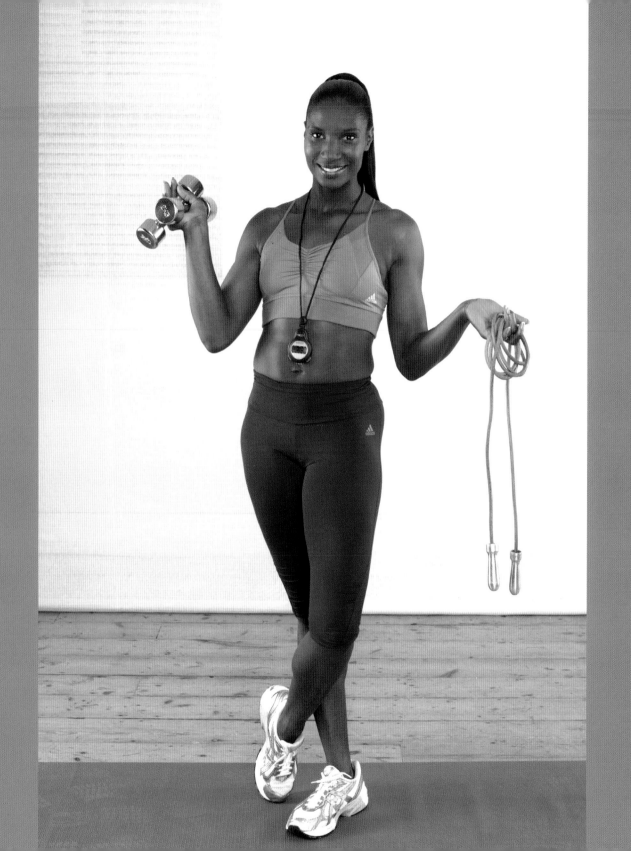

The Flat Tummy

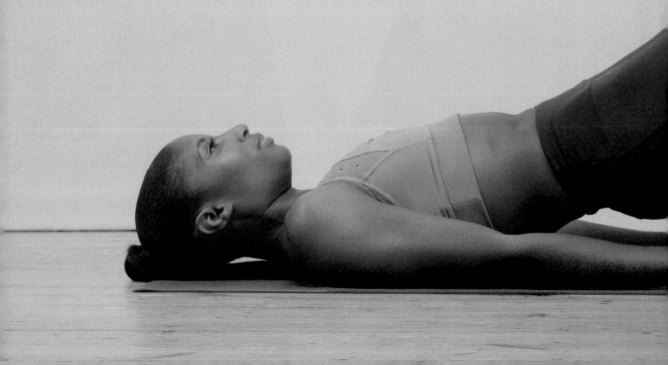

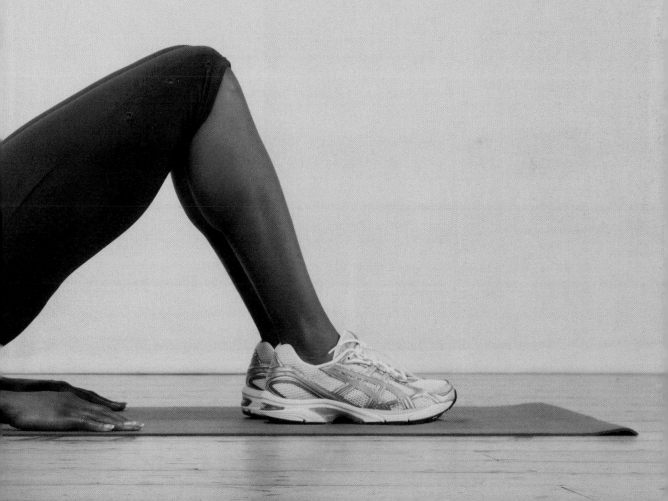

'OK, here we go! This chapter describes my flat tummy workout from warm up and stretches through to cool down. At the end of it, you will find programmes tailored to suit all fitness leves from beginner to adavnced.'

The Flat Tummy

Whatever your fitness level, the aim of this book is to give you the best possible workout in the shortest possible time. To see real results all you need to do is set aside half an hour, three times a week. You don't even need to go waste time going to the gym as all the exercises are designed to be done at home.

The exercises I've selected will work your abdominal muscles or 'abs' as they are more commonly referred to. Most people think that to get a flat stomach you just have to work on your 'six pack'. But to get the best flat tummy, you need to engage a broader set of muscles. To keep things simple, I have grouped the abs into three muscle areas:

The Front Muscle

People call this the 'six pack', but it really is one large muscle called the rectus abdominus.

The Side Muscles

Known as the obliques, which are engaged when you bend side to side.

The Deep Muscles

This is a section of muscle tissue deep in your tummy that holds everything together. Collectively, they are known as the transverse muscles. Try coughing to feel them being activated.

All of these muscles must be addressed in a complete abs programme. The Deep Muscles are especially important. I find that tilting my pelvis slightly towards the ceiling before I start each exercise engages them and flattens the back, putting you into the correct position to begin with. This lessens the pressure you put on the lower back while you workout and enables you to get the most out of the exercises.

You will notice I have included some exercises for the back muscles. They share a special relationship with the stomach muscles and should not be neglected. When performing any abs exercise you're contracting the muscles, making them shorter and more compact, while the muscles in your back are lengthened. If left unchecked, this can threaten the whole body's stability. Adding a few back strengthening exercises keeps the balance in this vital area and helps maintain good posture.

Preparation for exercise is crucial, so the Flat Tummy workout is going to start with a dynamic warm up (pages 26-31) followed by some stretching (pages 32-39). Both are key elements in preparing the body for action, getting the muscles warm and flexible, while raising your heart rate and opening up your lungs.

Having warmed up, you move on to the core of the workout. Here are 29 exercises that will work on your tummy and back muscles – and a few more muscles for good measure. I'm recommending that you first get to know these exercises by practising them a few times before we put them together into a specific workout – plans that I will present in the final programmes section.

You'll be finishing your workout with a cool down (pages 100-105), gentle stretching exercises that prevent soreness in your muscles, and bring your heart rate and breathing down.

Finally, everything comes together in the Programmes section (pages 106-113). Here are my specific workouts, tailored to all fitness levels, for you to practise and enjoy!

As with all exercise it is important that you have a clean bill of health. If you are post-pregnant or recovering from any recent injuries, consult your doctor or physiotherapist before attempting the exercises in this book.

Dynamic Warm Up

Preparing the body for exercise is important no matter what time of day you choose to do it because without a decent warm up you run the risk of injury.

In order to get the best out of your workout you need to have warm muscles that are ready to perform the range of movements required. This will allow you to execute the exercises more effectively. So I prefer to do a total body warm up which is dynamic and increases blood flow to the muscles, raises your heart rate and opens up the lungs, telling your brain and body to get ready for action! This is also a quicker way of raising the body temperature so you don't have to do lots of stretching.

I've given you three options for the dynamic warm up, which I hope you will find fun and a little bit different to what you have tried before. They are:

- Jogging on the spot
- Skipping
- Side lunges

Try them all and see which one you prefer. When you have decided which warm up works best for you, you can find specific routines in the Programmes section on pages 106–113.

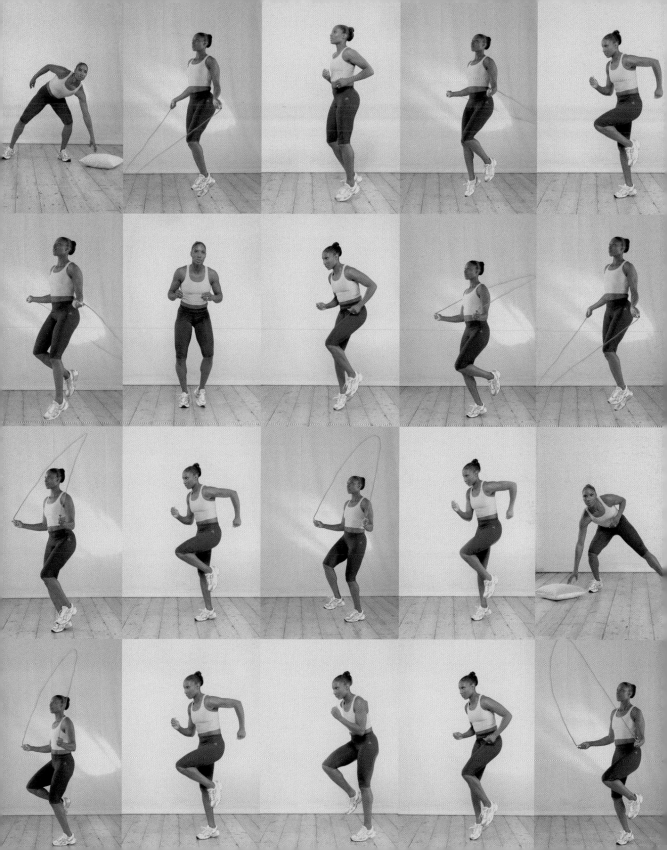

Jogging on the spot

Make sure you are wearing trainers
to support your feet and ankles,
then start off gently and find
your own rhythm.

TRAINING TIP
Remember to drop the shoulders
or think of keeping a long neck,
this will keep the tension out of
your shoulders.

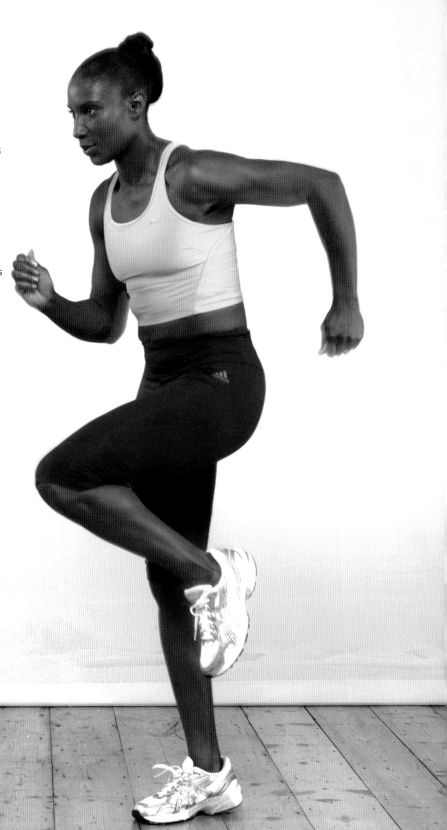

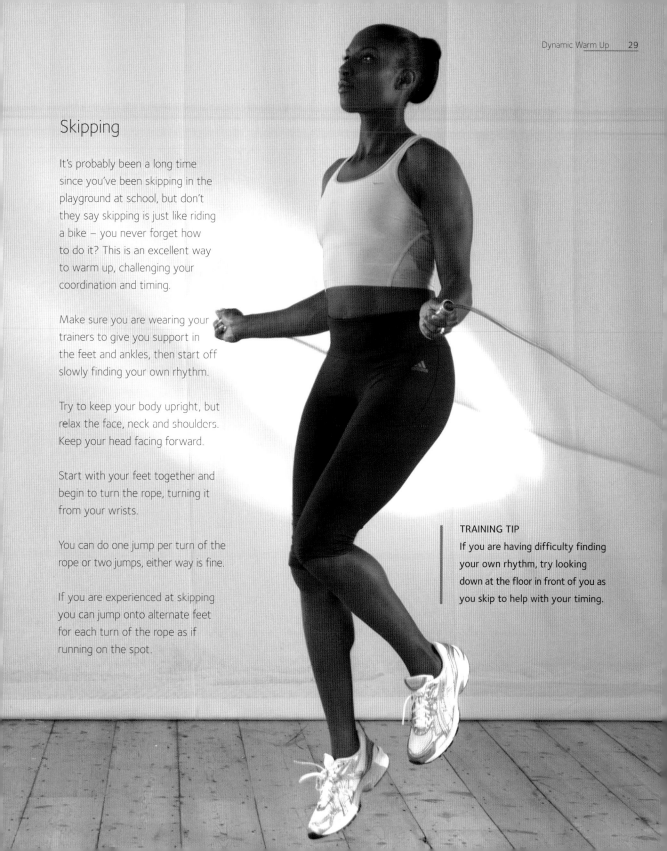

Skipping

It's probably been a long time since you've been skipping in the playground at school, but don't they say skipping is just like riding a bike – you never forget how to do it? This is an excellent way to warm up, challenging your coordination and timing.

Make sure you are wearing your trainers to give you support in the feet and ankles, then start off slowly finding your own rhythm.

Try to keep your body upright, but relax the face, neck and shoulders. Keep your head facing forward.

Start with your feet together and begin to turn the rope, turning it from your wrists.

You can do one jump per turn of the rope or two jumps, either way is fine.

If you are experienced at skipping you can jump onto alternate feet for each turn of the rope as if running on the spot.

TRAINING TIP
If you are having difficulty finding your own rhythm, try looking down at the floor in front of you as you skip to help with your timing.

Side lunges

Place two cushions approximately two metres (two large steps) apart and position yourself in the middle of them.

Take a side step to the right, then lunge forward with your body and touch the cushion with the fingers of your right hand.

Return to an upright position then repeat on the left side.

TRAINING TIP
Start off nice and slowly until you find your own range of movement. Don't worry if you can't reach the cushion at the beginning, once you've warmed up you can stretch a little further each time until you touch it.

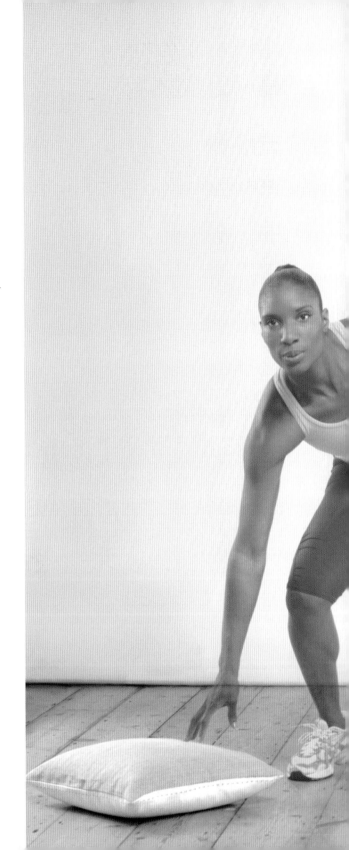

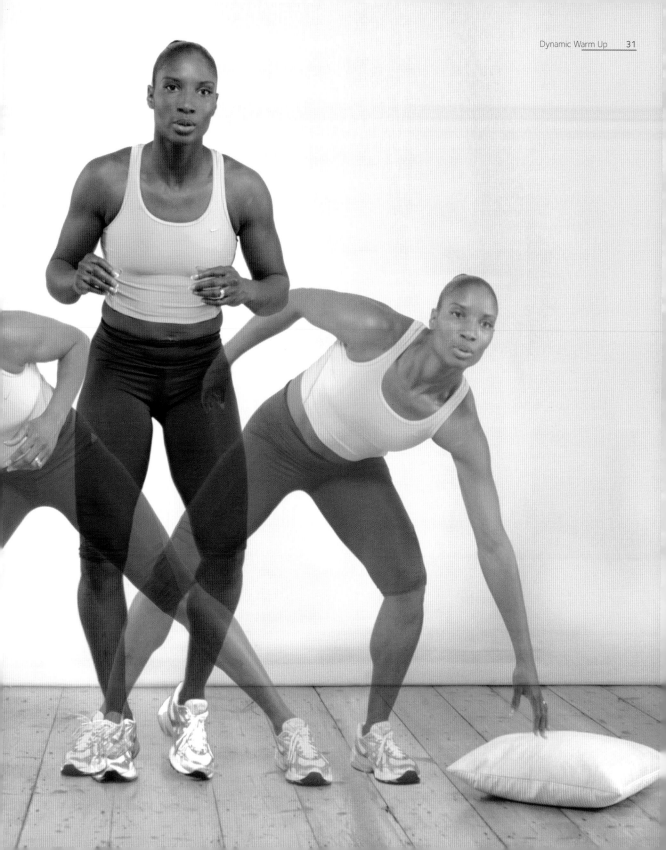

Stretching

Having kick started your body with the dynamic exercises the blood flow to your muscles will have increased making them warm and better prepared for the next stage which is stretching.

This is an important part of the warming up process as it encourages your muscles to lengthen and therefore increases your range of movement and flexibility.

Because this book is about how to manage the little time you have to exercise, this stretching routine should take you no longer than 5 minutes and targets the areas you will be specifically using for the exercises.

Stretching should be performed in a smooth and controlled manner to prevent any risk of injury to the muscles.

All these stretches should be repeated two or three times per exercise.

Side Stretch

1   Stand with your feet shoulder width apart.

2   Raise your left arm above your head and bend to
     the right. Hold for 5 seconds. You can rest your
     right hand on your hip for support. Return to
     upright position.

3   Change arms and repeat on the other side.

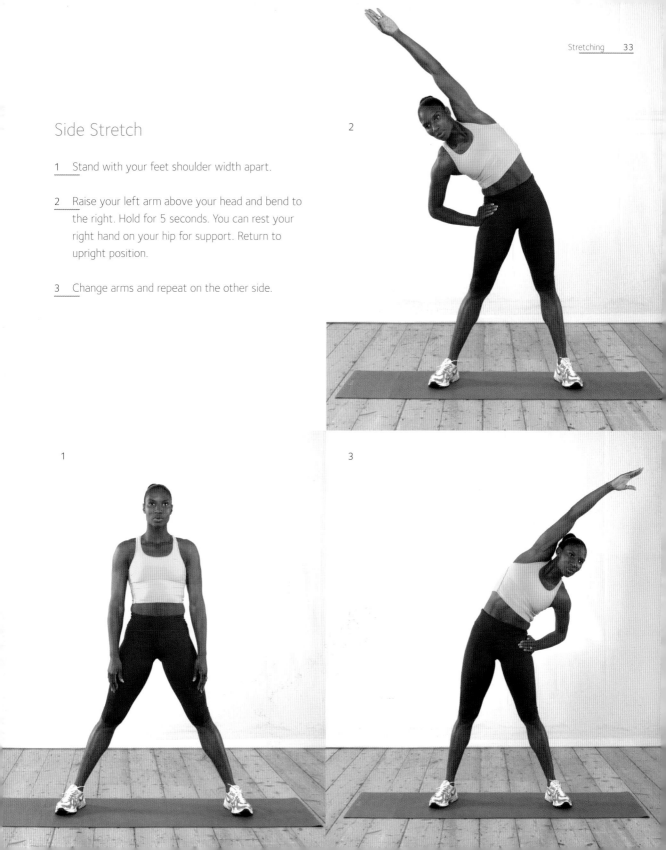

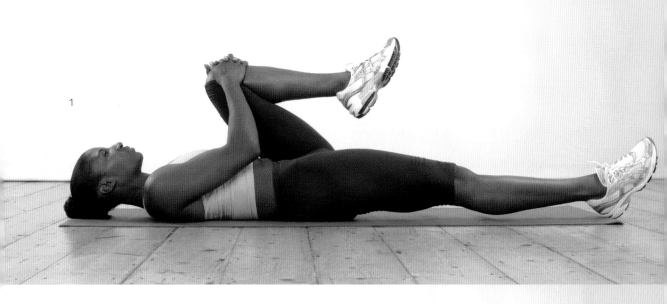

1

Glute (Bum) Stretch

1   Lie on your back, feet together. Raise your left
    knee and with your hands lightly clasped around
    it, pull it gently towards your chest. Hold for
    5 seconds.

2   Return to the starting position and repeat with
    the right knee.

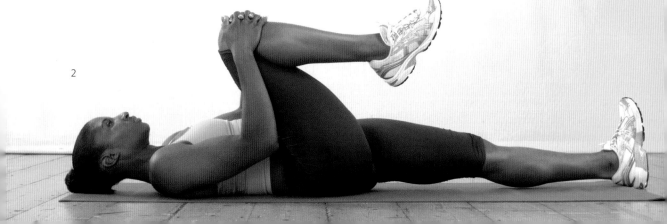

2

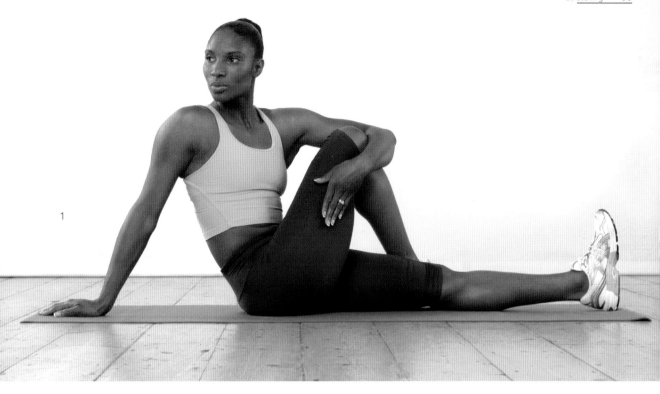

Glute and Side Stretch

Sit down with your legs together straight in front of you.

1   Bend your right knee and step the foot over the left leg. Take your right hand behind you for support and place your left hand on your right knee to hold it in position. Gently rotate your upper body as far as you can, looking over your right shoulder. Hold for 5 seconds.

2   Release and repeat to the left.

Lower Back Stretch

1   Lie on your back, arms out
    to the sides. Bend your left
    knee upwards, keeping your
    shoulders flat to the floor.

2   Lower the knee to the floor
    (or as far as you can go) to
    the right side and hold for 5
    seconds. You can place your
    right hand on your knee to
    keep it in position.

3   Release and return knee back to
    centre. Repeat on the left side.

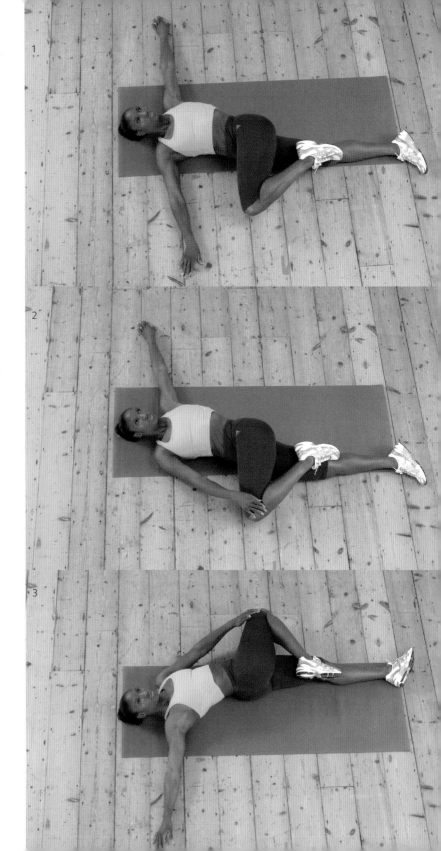

Side Stretch

1   Lie on your back, arms out to
    the sides. Bend your knees with
    your feet flat on the floor.

2   Keeping your shoulders flat
    to the floor and your head
    straight, lower both knees
    to the right and hold for
    5 seconds.

3   Release and return both knees
    to the centre, then repeat to
    the left.

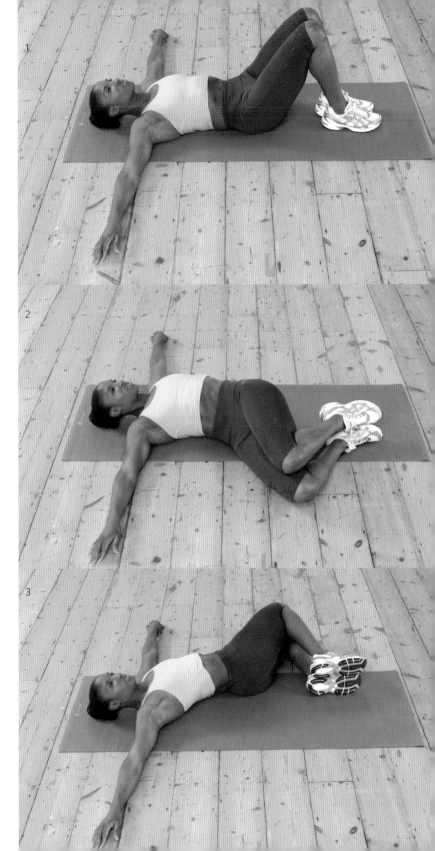

Calf Stretch

Stand with feet together and step
your left foot forward. Bend your
left knee, but keep your right leg
straight and your heel in contact
with the floor. Rest your hands on
your left thigh for support. Hold
for 5 seconds and repeat on the
other side.

Hamstring Stretch

Step your left foot forward and
lean your torso over it, bending
your right knee as you do so. Keep
bending forward until you feel the
stretch at the back of your left leg.
Hold for 5 seconds and repeat on
the other side.

Side Twist

Raise your arms to shoulder height
elbows facing out and smoothly
twist your upper body to the right
side, keeping your pelvis facing
forwards as you do so. Return to
centre, then twist to the left.

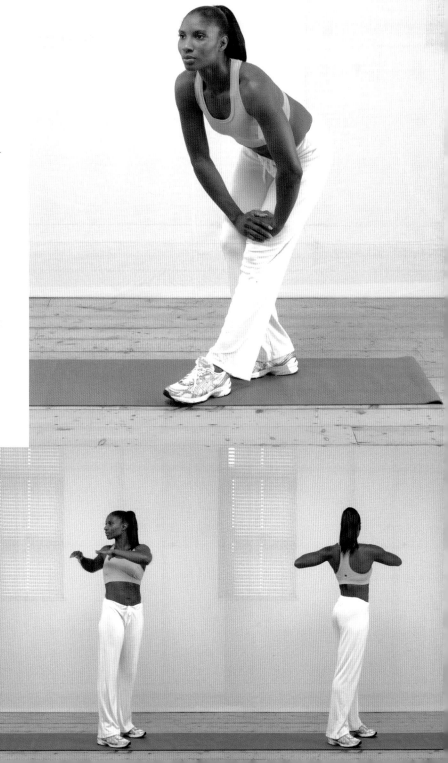

The Exercises

Having warmed up and stretched, you're now ready to begin the exercises themselves. In the following pages, there are 29 exercises for your tummy and back muscles. I have shown all the exercises with step-by-step instructions on how to do them, but you'll have to wait until the Programmes section (pages 106-113) before you can put them together into a specific workout. Before you get there though, you should perform each exercise three or four times on two non-consecutive days. This should help programme your brain, letting you automatically find the right positions and make the right movements without having to keep referring back to the book.

Try to get as close as possible to the pictures you see, but remember to take it easy and start off slowly so you can find a rhythm that suits you. The emphasis is always on control, not speed. Focusing on your breathing – inhaling and exhaling correctly – will help you keep a consistent tempo while you perform each exercise and energise your muscles by giving them a fresh supply of oxygen.

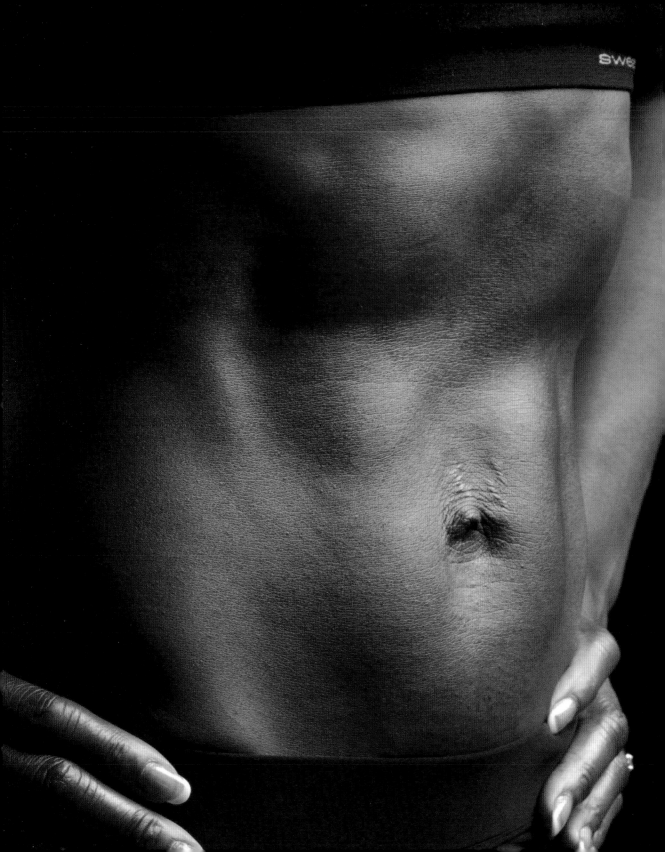

Knee Lifts

For the Front and Deep muscles

1   Lie flat on the floor, with your legs straight, hands behind your head.

2   Keep your left leg straight and your back nice and flat and raise your right knee bent at a ninety-degree angle, toes pointing towards the ceiling.

3   Return your right leg to the starting position, then repeat raising your left leg.

> TRAINING TIP
> Tilt your pelvis towards the ceiling, and maintain the tilt throughout the exercise.

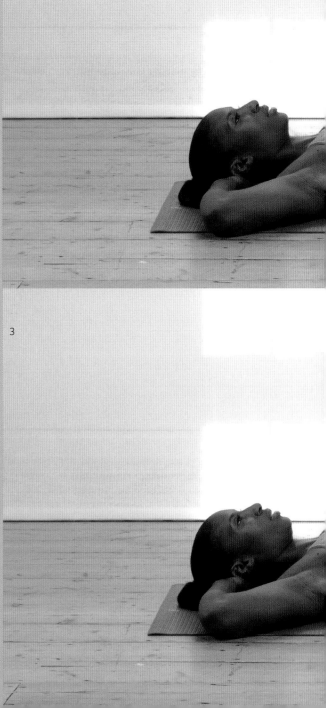

2

3

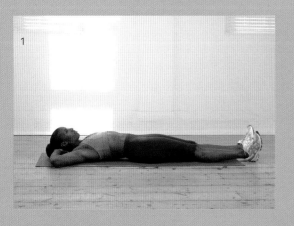

1

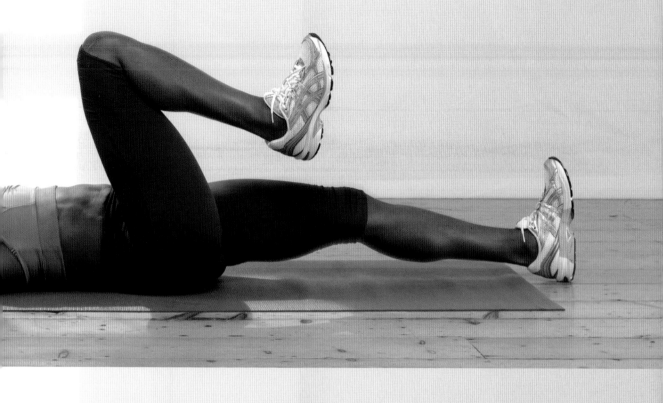

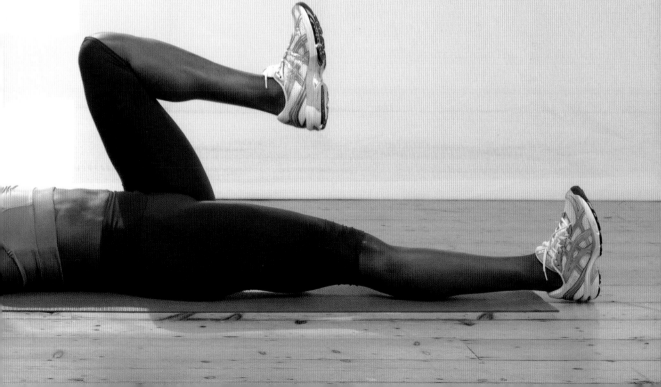

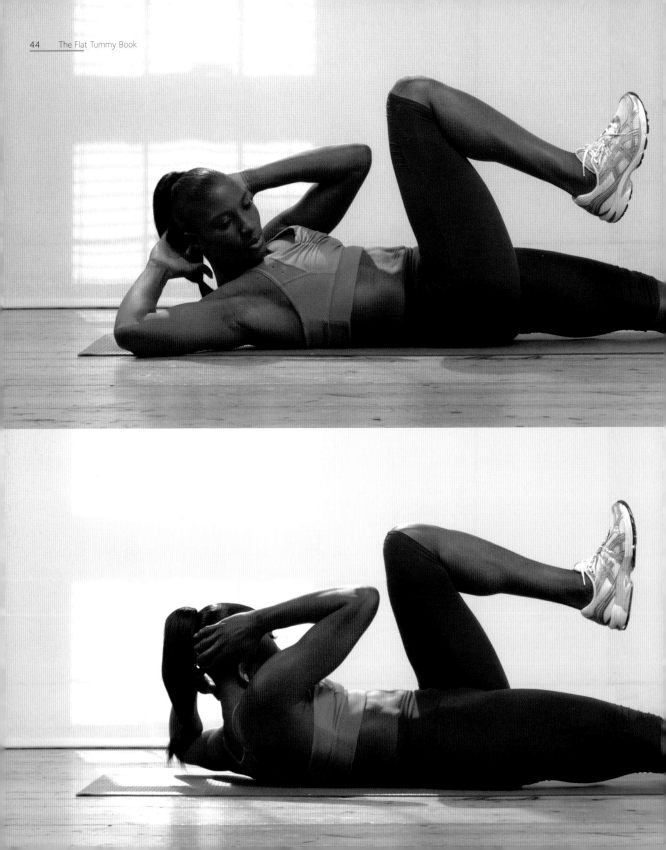

2

Advanced Knee Lifts

For the Front and Deep muscles

1   Lie flat on the floor, with your legs straight, hands behind your head.

2   Keep your left leg straight and raise your right knee bent at a ninety-degree angle. At the same time rotate your upper body so that your left elbow moves towards your right knee. Return to the starting position.

3   Raise your left leg to the same position and repeat with your right elbow.

TRAINING TIP
Tilt your pelvis towards the ceiling, and maintain the tilt throughout the exercise.

3

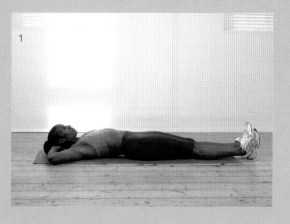

1

Bicycle

For the Front and Deep muscles

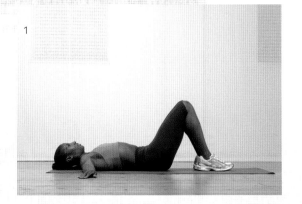

1   Lie on your back, arms out to the sides, palms flat
    on the floor, knees bent.

2   Draw your knees up towards the ceiling.

3   Begin to pedal as if you are on an imaginary bicycle.
    Keep your back flat and make big, complete circles
    with your feet. Make sure that the bottom of the
    circle is close to the floor.

> TRAINING TIP
> At the bottom of your pedal stroke, your feet should
> be as near to the end of your exercise mat as you can
> manage. Imagine you are trying to push the pedals as
> far away from you as possible.

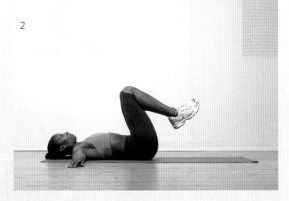

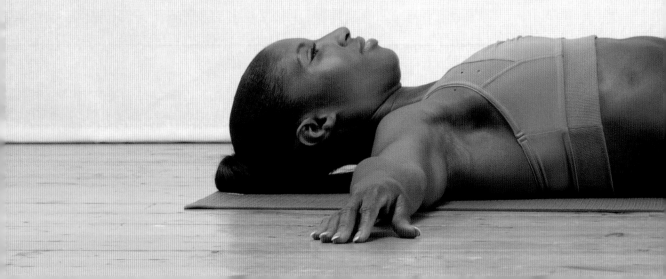

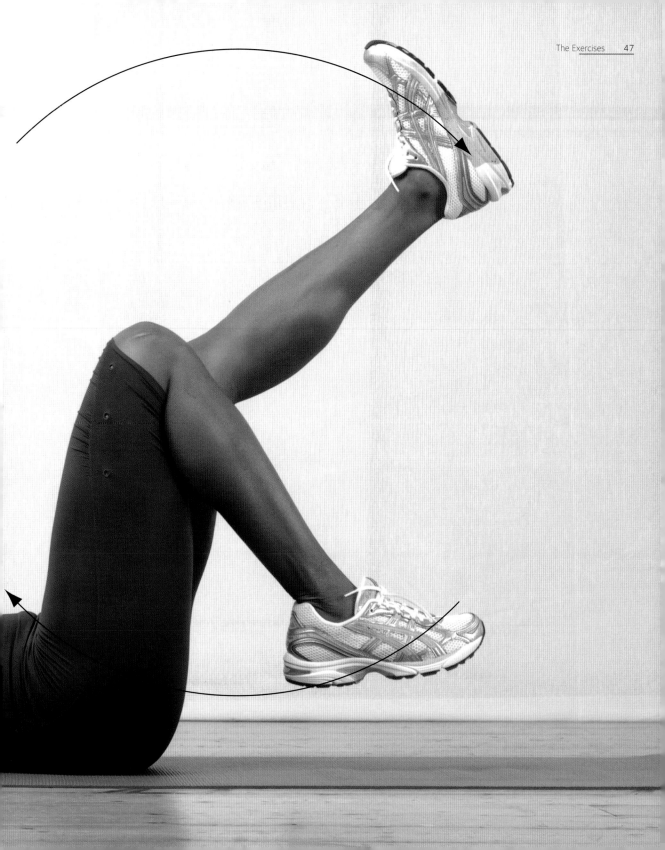

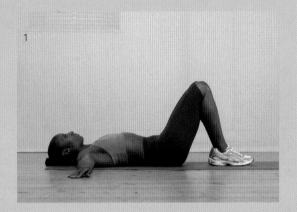

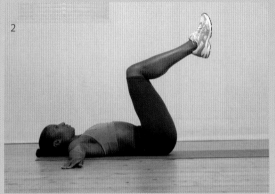

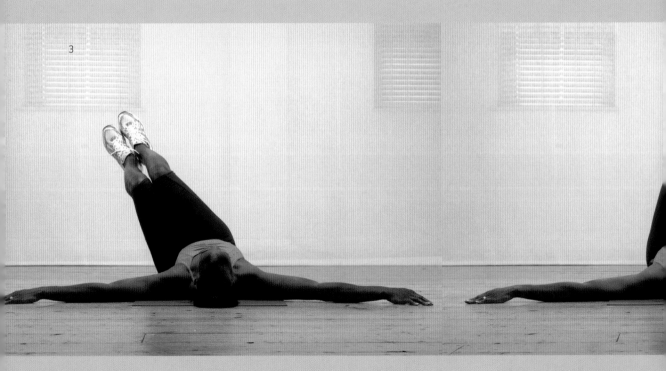

Bent Knee Wipers

For the Front, Side and Deep muscles

1 Lie on your back arms out to the sides, palms flat on the floor, knees bent.

2 Keep the small of your back flat to the floor and raise your knees towards the ceiling to a ninety-degree angle. Your ankles and feet are together.

3 Lower your legs to the side from the hips to about a forty-five degree angle. Return to centre and repeat on the other side.

If you are uncomfortable in this position, you can place a towel under your buttocks to give your pelvic bone extra cushioning (below).

TRAINING TIP
Tilt your pelvis towards the ceiling, and maintain the tilt throughout the exercise.

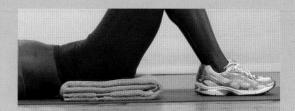

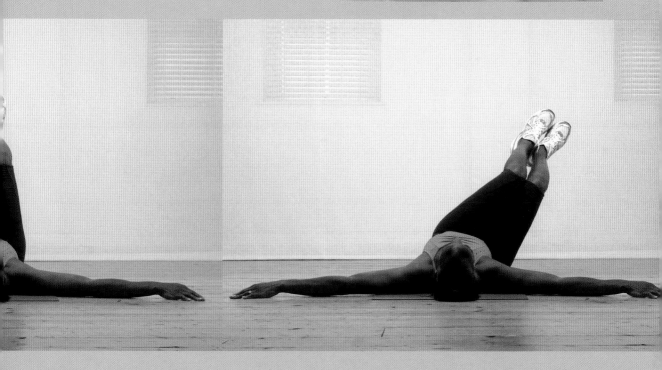

Straight Leg Wipers

For the Front, Side and Deep muscles

1   Lie on your back, arms out to the sides, legs bent with knees and feet together.

2   Raise your legs into the air, keeping your knees slightly bent.

3   Rotate your legs from the hips to the right – go as far as you can without lifting your shoulders from the floor.

4   Return your legs to the centre and repeat to the left – like windscreen wipers.

TRAINING TIP
Tilt your pelvis towards the ceiling, and maintain the tilt throughout the exercise.

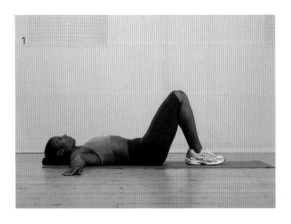

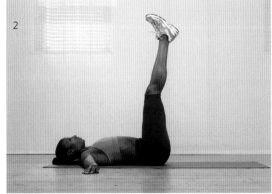

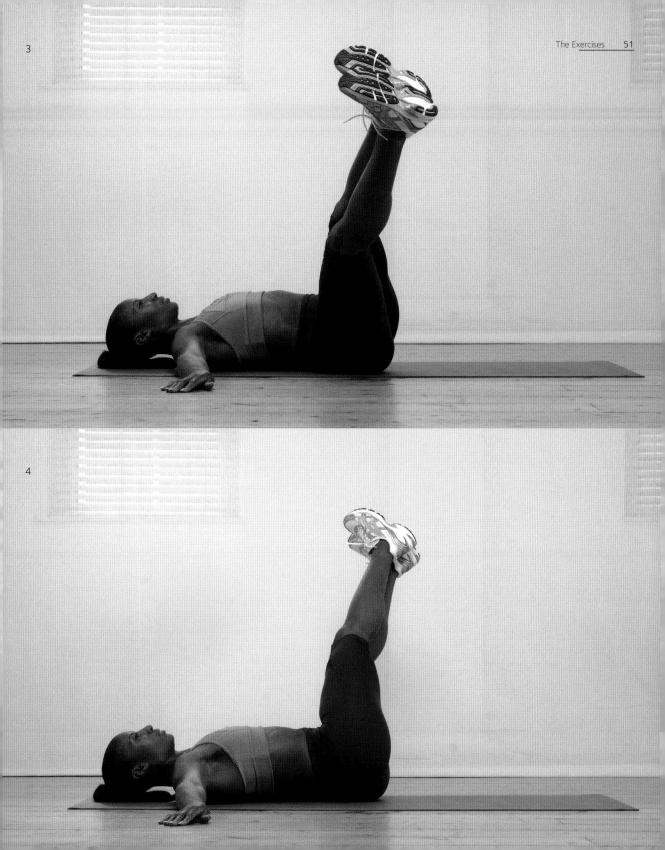

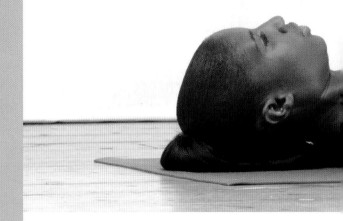

1

Open/Close Knees

For the Front and Deep muscles

1   Lie on your back with your legs together, knees bent
    and feet flat on the floor.

2   Put your fingers under the small of your back either
    side, so that your back squashes them. This makes
    sure that your back is flat.

3   Let your knees fall apart as far as you can go, then
    close them and repeat, maintaining the pressure on
    your fingers.

3

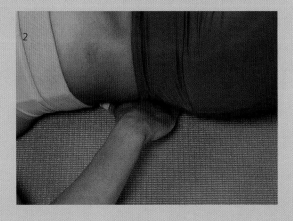

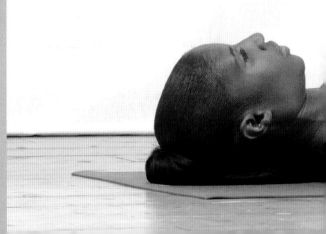

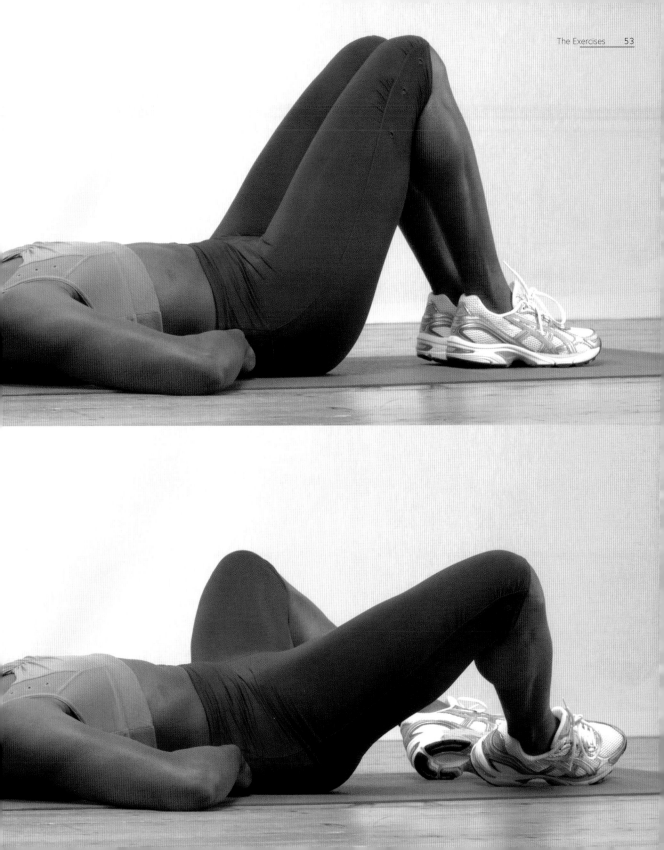

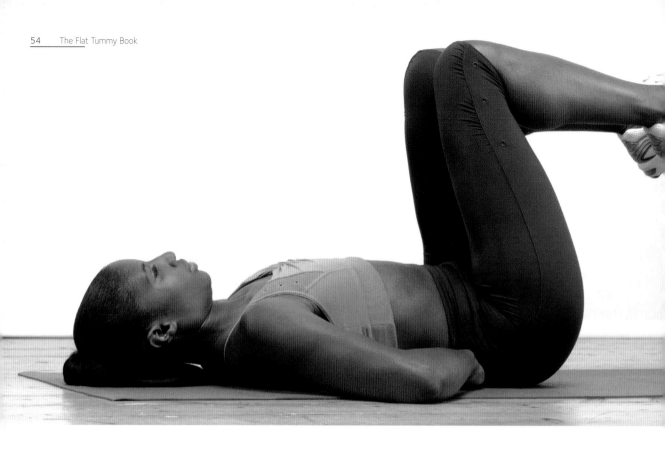

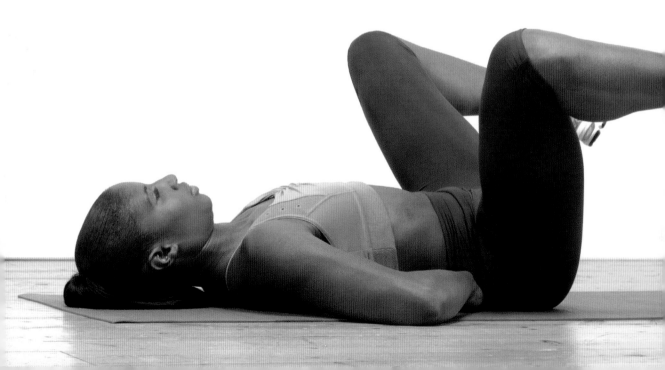

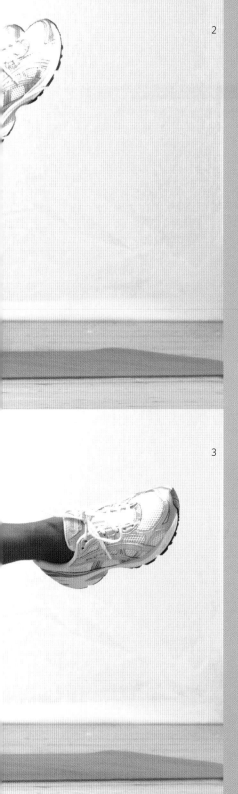

Advanced Open/Close Knees

For the Front and Deep muscles

1   Lie on your back with your legs together, knees bent and feet flat on the floor. Put your fingers under the small of your back either side, so that your back squashes them, making sure that your back is flat (see p.52).

2   Raise your knees towards the ceiling to a ninety-degree angle.

3   Open your knees and feet as far as they can go.

Close them and then lower your feet back to the starting position and repeat.

TRAINING TIP
Remember to keep returning your feet back to the starting position and to keep squashing your fingers.

3

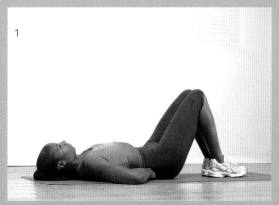

1

Upper Trunk Rotations

For the Front, Side and Deep muscles

1   Lie on your right side with your knees bent at a
    ninety-degree angle, knees and feet together. Make
    sure you are lying straight. Tighten your stomach
    and buttocks and clasp your hands gently behind
    your head. Close your elbows in front of your face.

2   Rotate your upper body towards the left, open your
    elbows as far as you can, aiming to get your left
    elbow as close to the floor as possible.

Turn over onto your left side and repeat the
exercise.

TRAINING TIP
For comfort, you can place a towel or small
cushion under your hipbone.

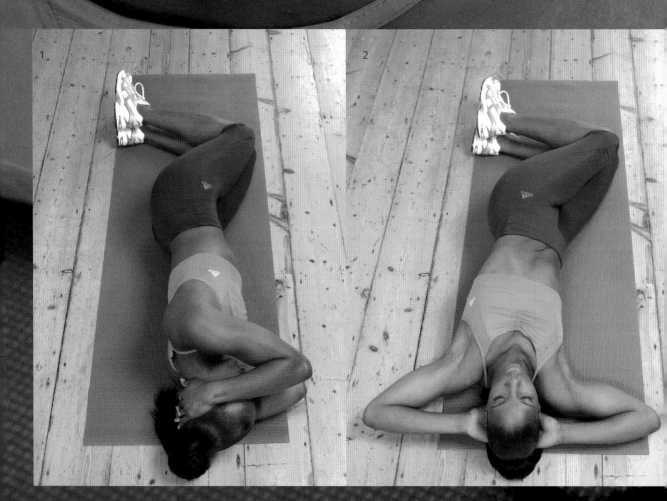

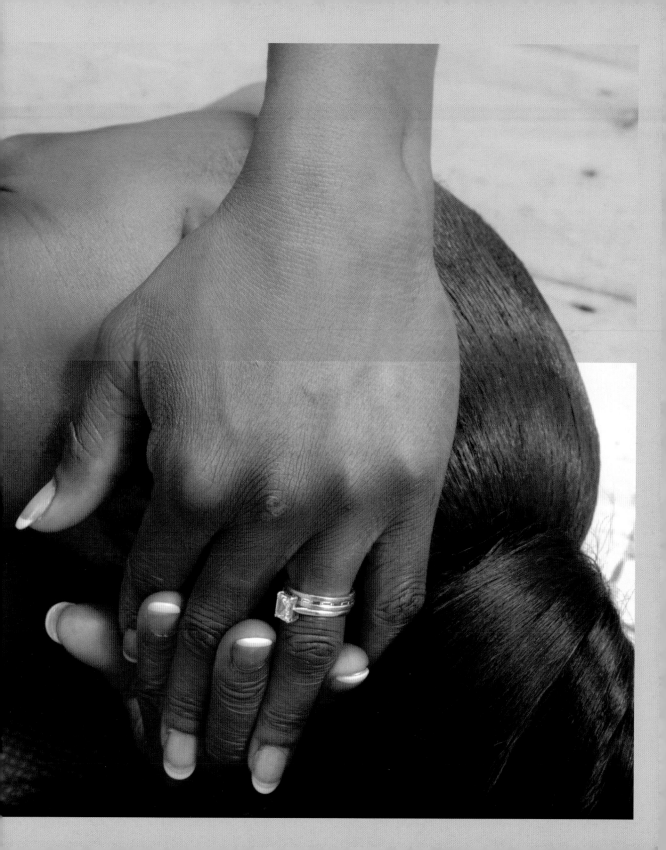

Leg Rotations

For the Side and Deep muscles

1   Lie on your right side, your knees bent together on the floor. Straighten your right arm underneath your head. Place your left hand on the floor in front of your body to act as a stabiliser. Keep your tummy tucked in.

2   Keep your knees together and rotate them towards the ceiling at forty-five degrees, keeping your upper body still. Return knees to the floor.

Turn over onto your left side and repeat the exercise.

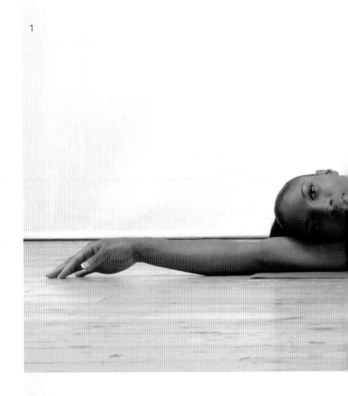

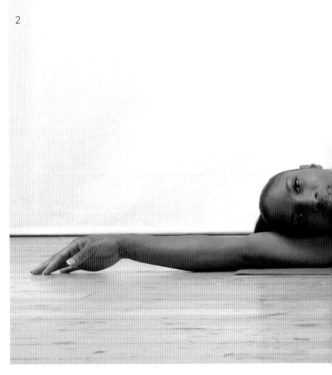

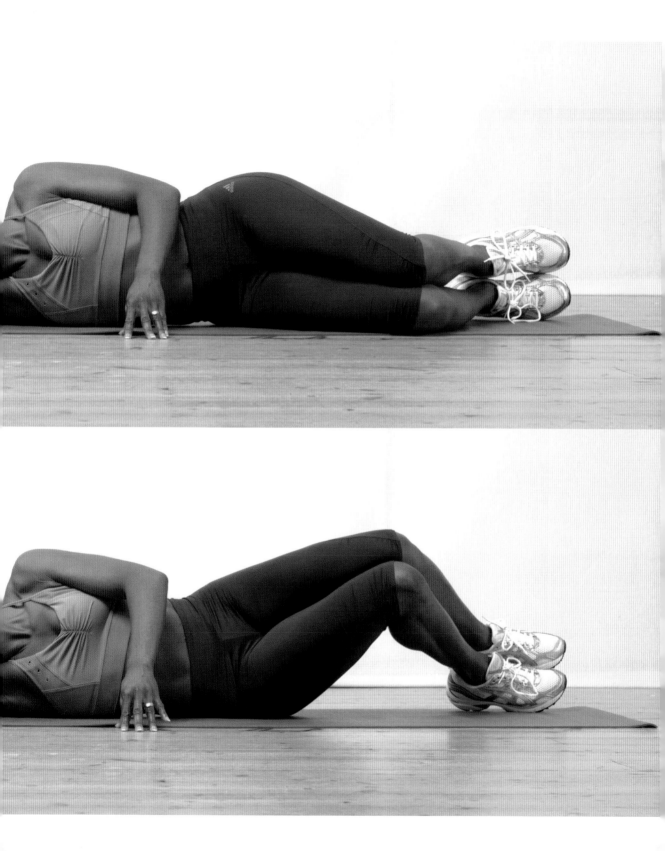

Straight Leg Lifts

For the Side muscles

1   Lie on your right side, legs straight. Straighten your
    right arm underneath your head. Keep your body
    nice and straight and place your left hand on the
    floor in front of you to give stability.

2   Raise your left leg in line with your body to about
    thirty degrees. Keep your tummy tucked in and
    squeeze your buttocks. This will help to keep
    your body straight.

    Repeat, lying on the other side.

    NOTE
    This exercise will also engage your glutes.

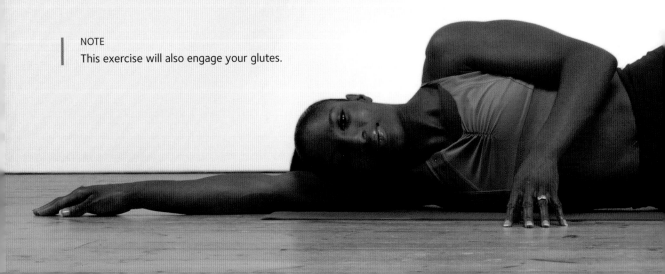

1

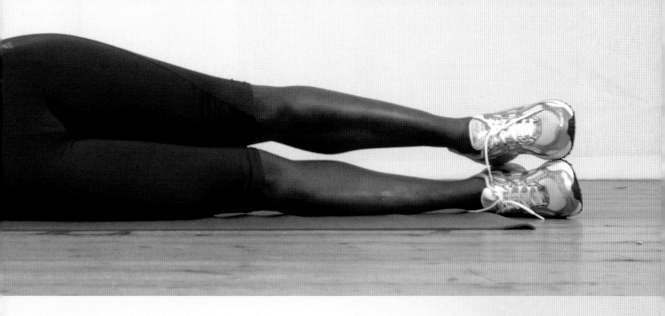

2

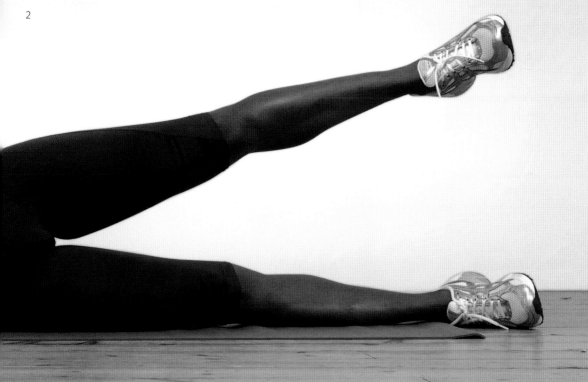

Advanced Straight Leg Lifts

For the Side muscles

1   Lie on your right side, legs straight. Straighten your
    right arm underneath your head. Keep your body
    nice and straight and place your left hand on the
    floor in front of you to give stability.

2   Keeping your ankles together, lift them slightly (about
    ten inches) off the floor. Keep your tummy tucked
    in and squeeze your buttocks.

    Repeat, lying on the other side.

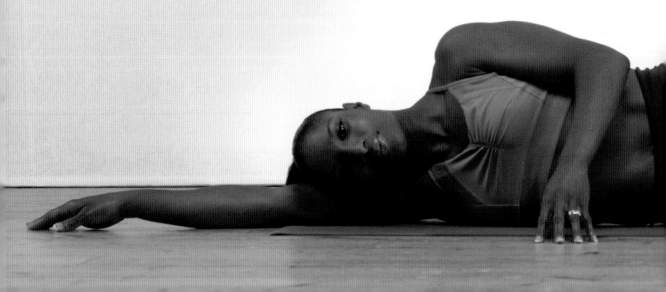

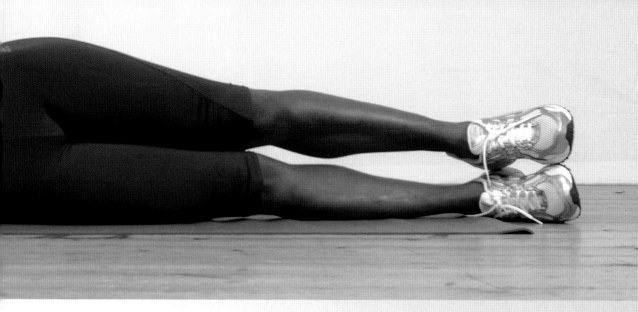

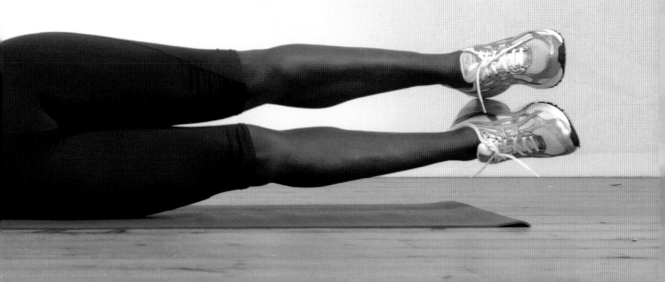

Seated Floor Touches

For the Front, Side and Deep muscles

1   Sit on the floor, knees bent and slightly apart. Your heels are on the floor, toes pointing up to the ceiling.

2   Lean back to a forty-five degree angle, keeping your back firm.

3   Raise your arms above your head.

4   Then in a fluid movement touch the floor on your right side with your fingertips of both hands.

5   Bring your arms back over your head to touch the floor on the left side and repeat.

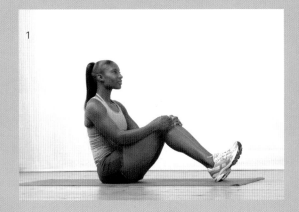

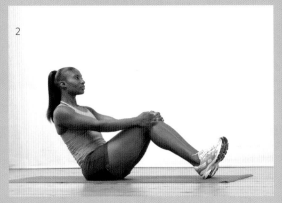

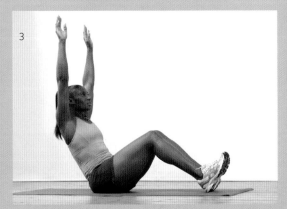

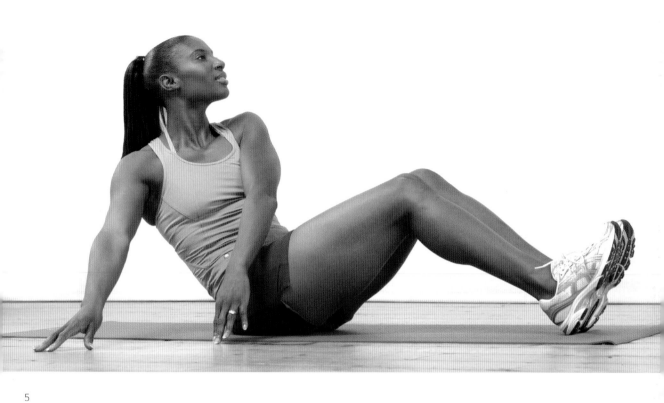

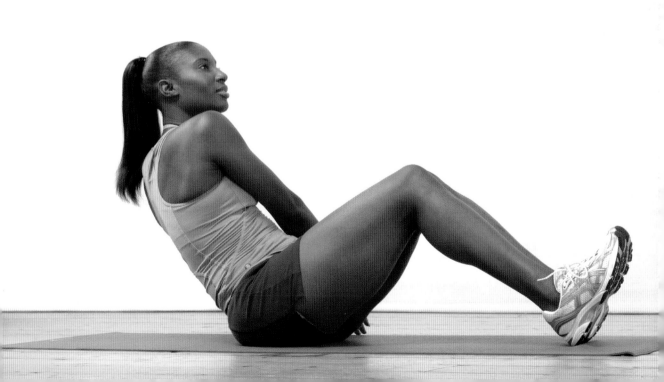

Intermediate Floor Touches

For the Front, Side and Deep muscles

You will need a 2 kilo weight for this exercise.

1   Sit on the floor, knees bent and slightly apart.
Your heels are on the floor, toes pointing up to
the ceiling. Lean back to a forty-five degree angle,
keeping your back firm. Take your weight in both
hands on your right side.

2   Lift the weight over your head.

3   Gently touch the floor with it on your left side.

Bring the weight back over your head to touch the
floor on the left side and repeat.

TRAINING TIP
**Try to keep your arms as straight as possible and
make the full arc.**

1

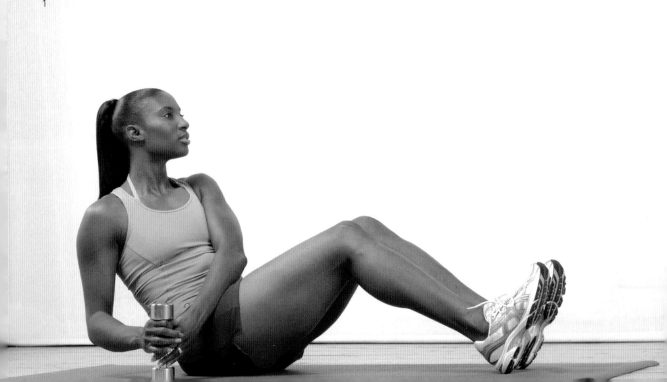

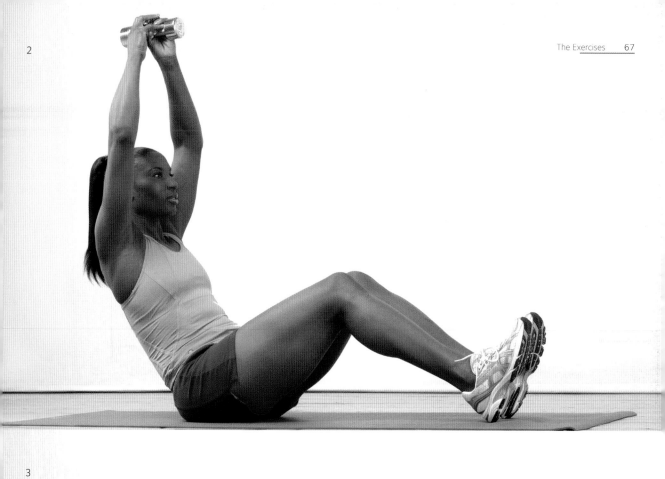

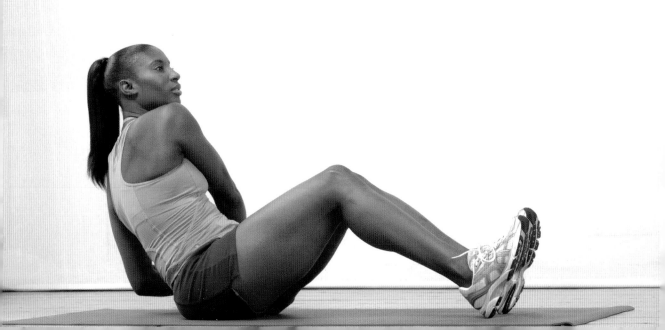

Advanced Floor Touches

For the Front, Side and Deep muscles

You will need a 2 kilo weight for this exercise.

1   Sit on the floor, knees bent and slightly apart. Your heels are on the floor, toes pointing up to the ceiling. Lean back to a forty-five degree angle, keeping your back firm. Take your weight in both hands on your right side.

2   Lift your heels off the floor and cross your ankles for stability.

3   Keeping your arms bent, move the weight over your stomach to your left side.

Bring the weight back over your stomach to your right side and reapeat.

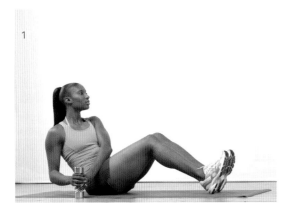

1

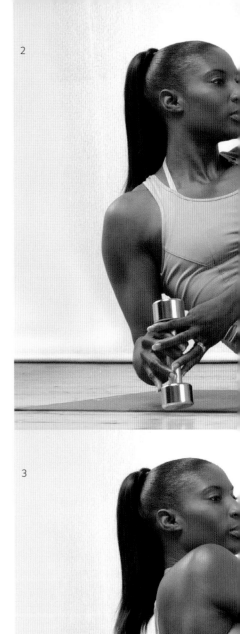

2

3

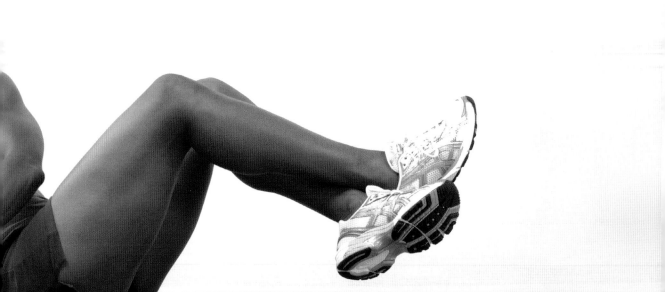

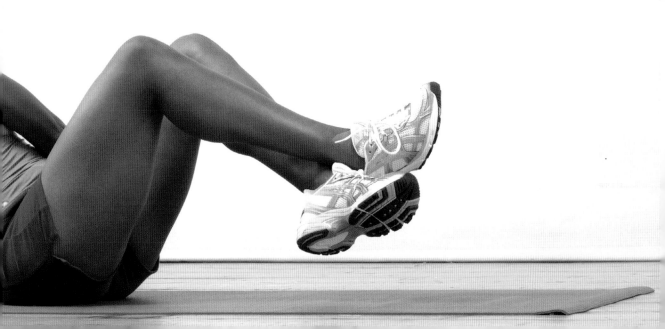

Seated Heel Touches

For the Front muscle

You will need a couple of cushions for this exercise.

1   Sit on the floor leaning back to a forty-five degree
    angle, with your arms behind you for support. Put
    your heels on the floor to the left side of the cushions.

2   Raise your right heel up and over the cushions.

3   Touch the floor on the other side, then return to
    the starting point. Repeat.

    Swap both feet over to the right side of the cushions
    and repeat the exercise with the left foot.

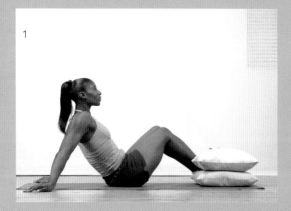

1

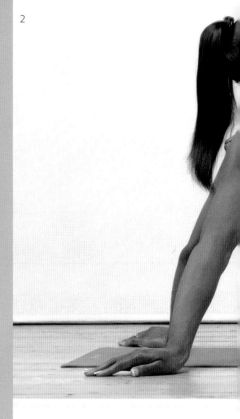

2

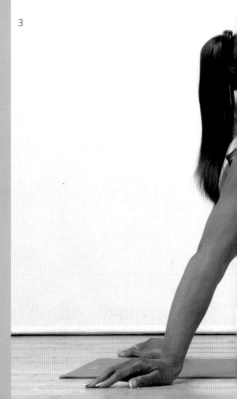

3

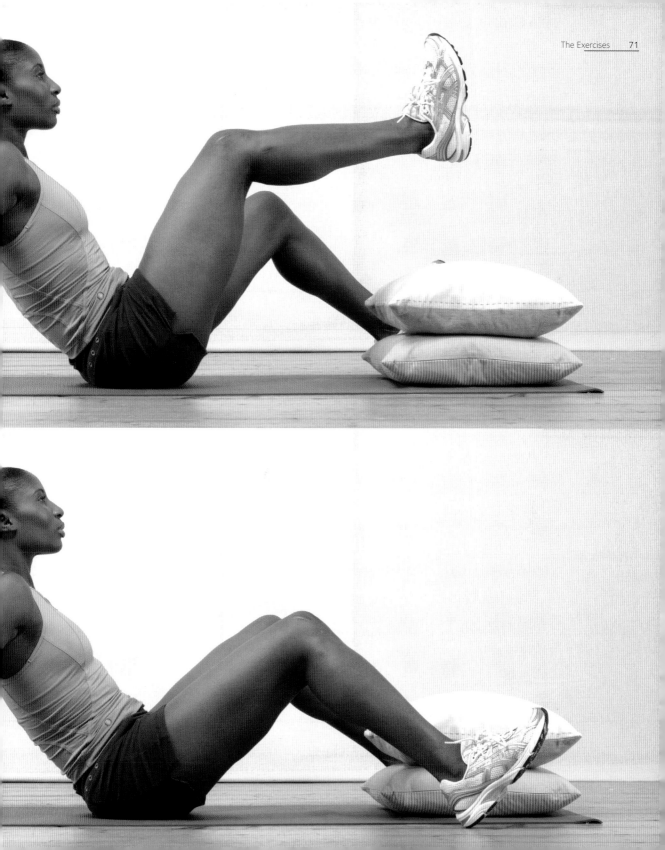

Advanced Seated Heel Touches

For the Front, Side and Deep muscles

You will need a couple of cushions for this exercise.

1   Sit on the floor leaning back to a forty-five degree angle, with your arms behind you for support. Put your heels on the floor to the left side of the cushions.

2   Lift both your heels up and over the cushions.

3   Touch the floor on the other side.

Return to the starting point and repeat.

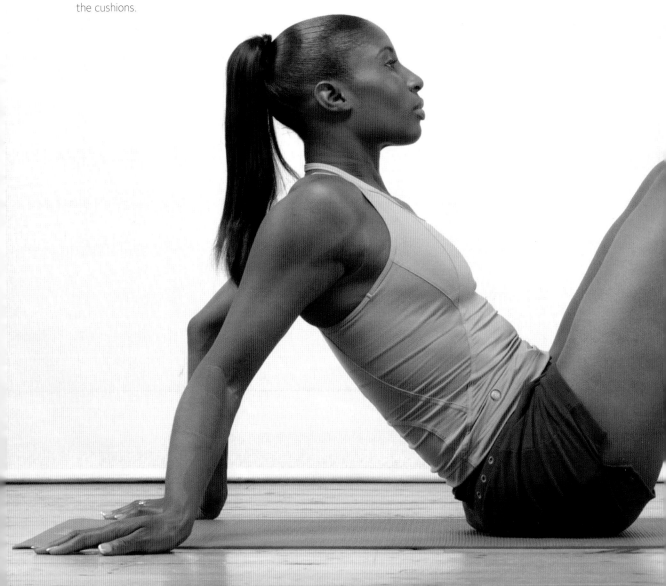

1

3

2

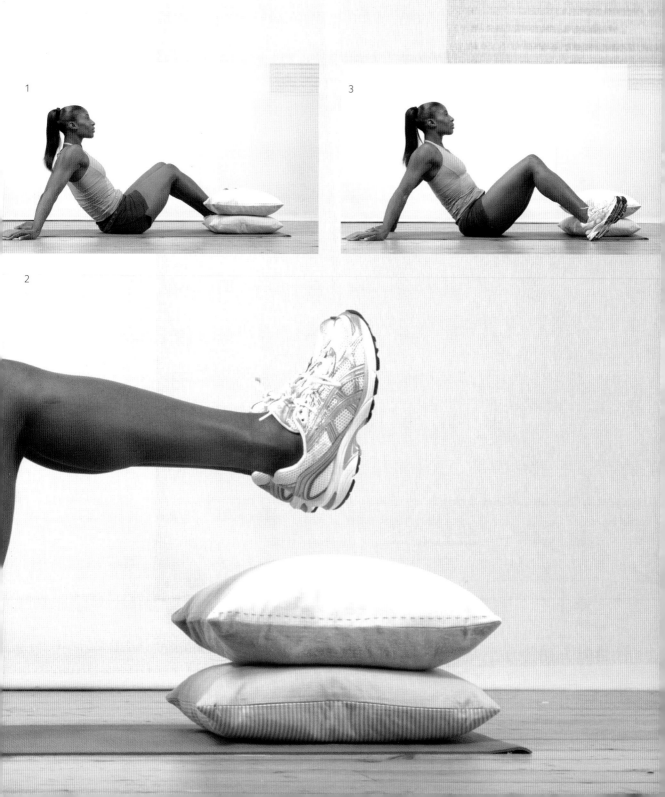

Kneeling Side Bends

For the Side muscles

1   Kneel on the floor with your knees hip-width apart.
    Put your hands behind your head with the fingers
    lightly clasped.

2   Bend your upper body sideways to the right
    towards the floor. Return to the centre and repeat
    a couple of times.

3   Then repeat the exercise to the left.

TRAINING TIP
Keep your tummy tucked in. Don't cheat the
movement by bending slightly forward.

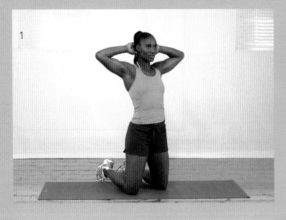

2

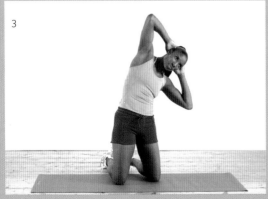

1

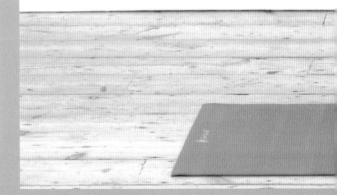

3

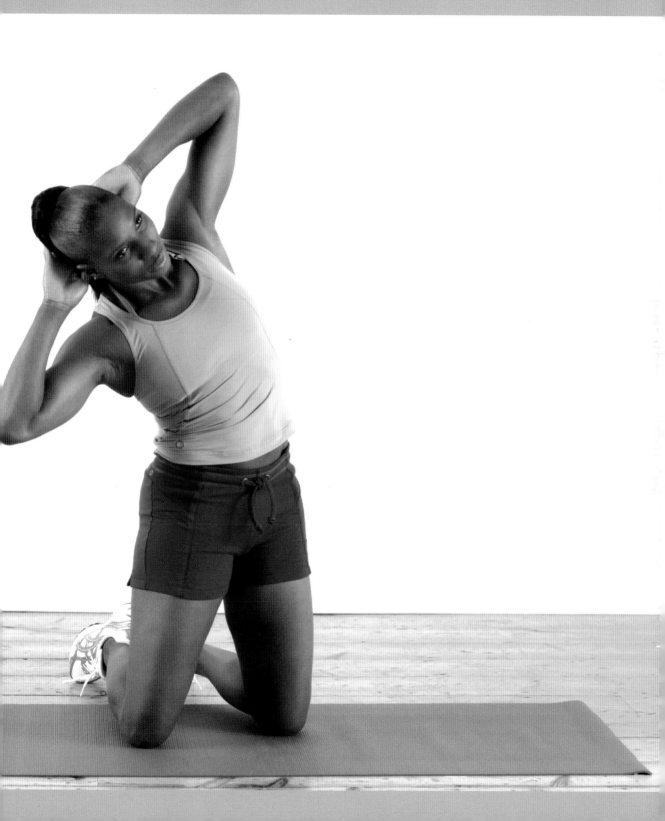

2   1

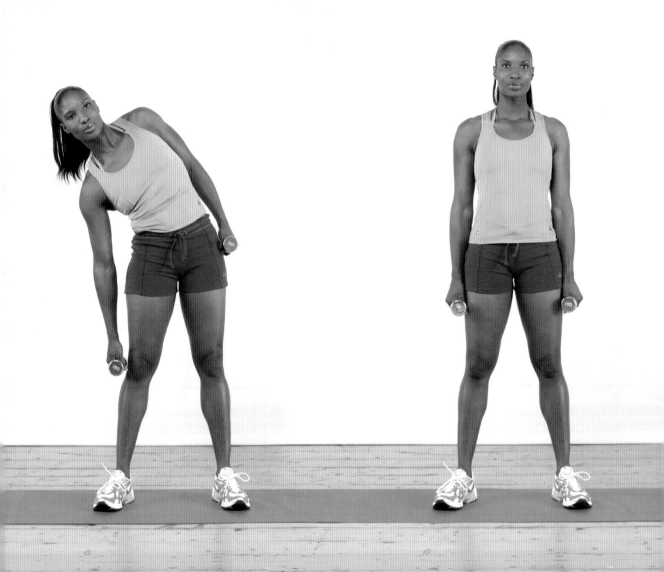

Intermediate Side Bends

For the Side muscles

3

You will need your weight for this exercise.

1   Stand with your feet shoulder-width apart.
Hold your weight in each hand.

2   Bend to the right in a fluid movement, reaching
down with your right hand as you do so.

Return to the centre and take a slight pause.

3   Then bend to your left side, reaching down with
your left hand.

TRAINING TIP
Don't over-stretch. Work within your own range
of movement.

Advanced Side Bends

For the Side muscles

You will need your weight for this exercise.

1   Stand with your feet shoulder-width apart. Hold your weight in both hands above your head, arms straight. Keep your tummy tucked in.

2   Turn your torso to the right.

3   Keeping your arms straight and bending your knees, lower the weight to touch your right knee.

Return to start position (figure 1).

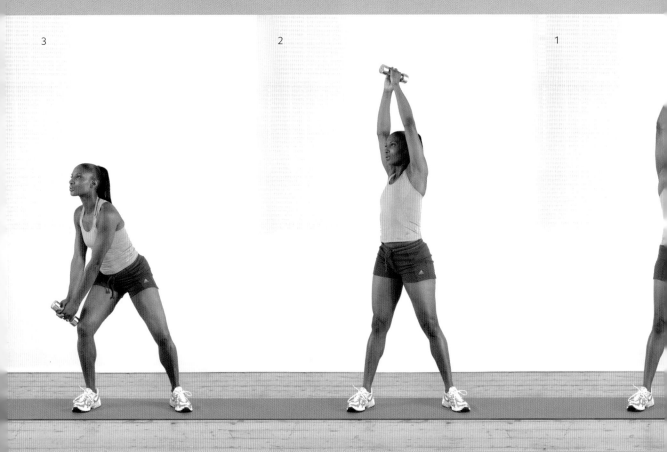

4   Turn your torso to the left.

5   Keeping your arms straight and bending your knees,
     lower the weight to touch your left knee.

     Return to start position (figure 1) and repeat.

4

5

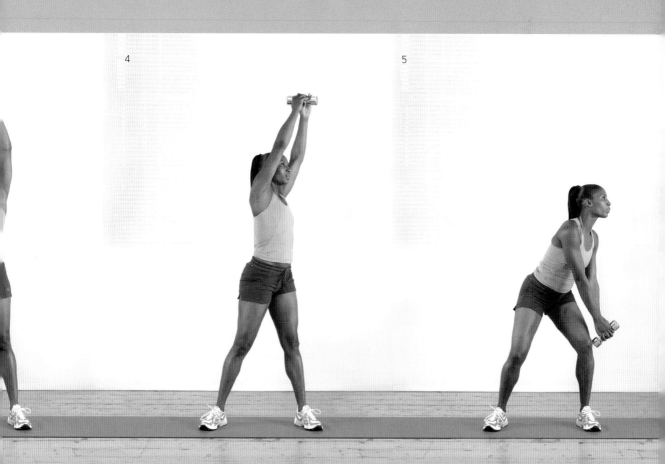

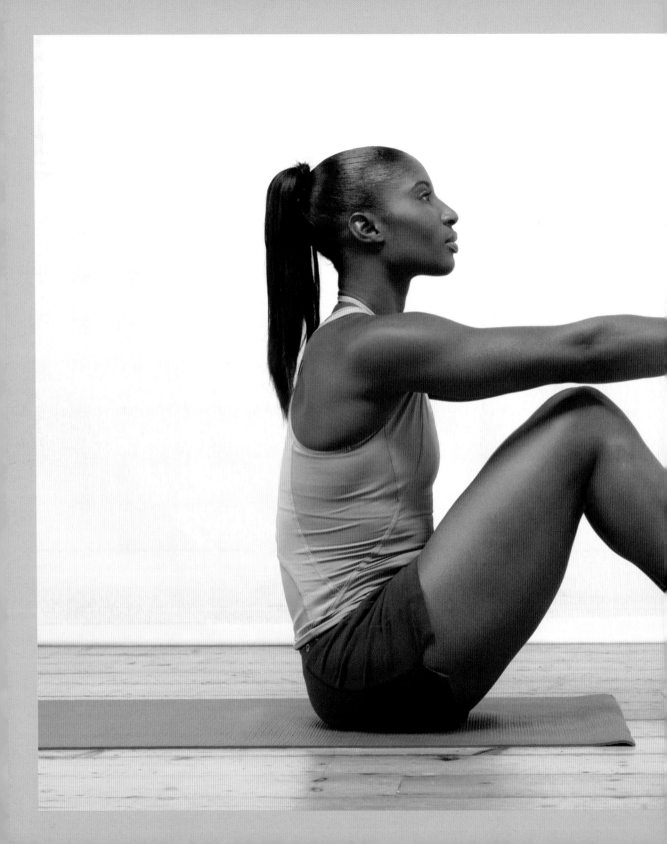

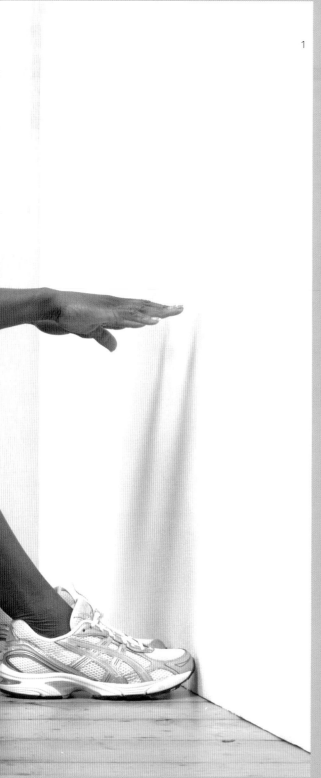

1

Seated Wall Touches

For the Front muscles

1   Sit facing a wall, knees slightly open and bent, with
     your toes touching the wall, arms straight in front
     of you.

2   Lean back to forty-five degrees, then lean forward
     to touch the wall with your fingertips, keeping tall
     through the spine.

     Repeat.

TRAINING TIP
**You can increase the difficulty of this exercise
by leaning back further.**

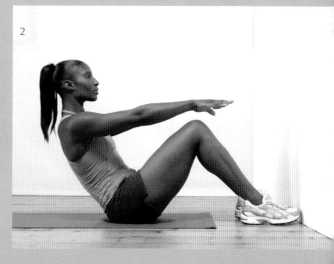

2

Simple Crunches

For the Front and Deep muscles

1   Lie on the floor with your hands behind your head.
    Tilt your pelvis towards the ceiling and maintain the
    tilt throughout the exercise. Raise your legs in the
    air slightly bent, feet crossed at the ankles.

2   Raise your head and shoulders, closing your elbows
    as you do so. Touch your chin to your chest and
    lower back to the floor.

    Repeat.

1

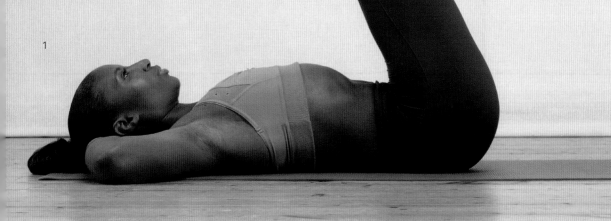

Avoid pulling on the back of your head with your hands.

2

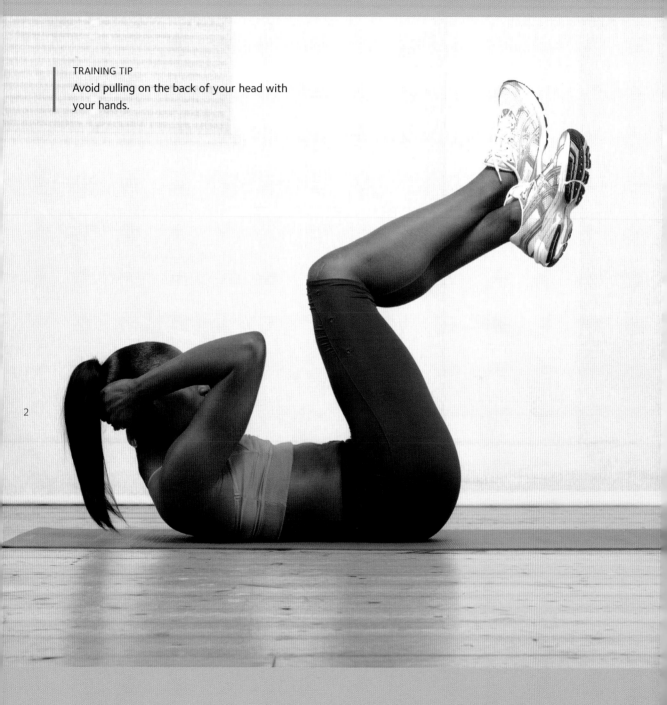

Hip Raise with Knee Lift

For the Side and Deep muscles

1   Lie on your back with your arms by your sides, palms
     down, your legs and feet together, knees bent.

2   Tighten your buttocks and lift your hips towards
     the ceiling.

3   Raise your right knee up and then put it down again.

4   Raise your left knee up and then put it down again.

     Repeat, as if walking on the spot.

TRAINING TIP
Try to keep your torso stable and don't drop
your hips. You will notice your buttocks working
as well.

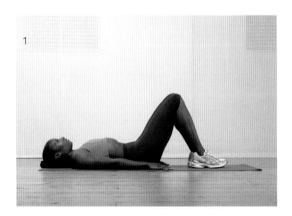

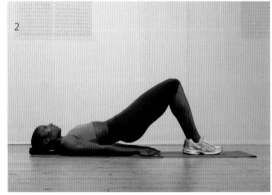

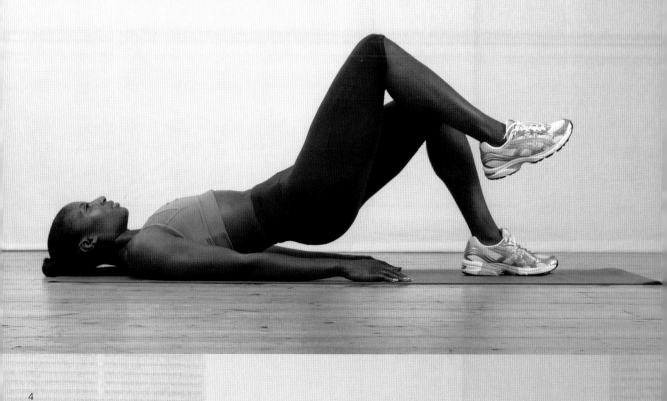

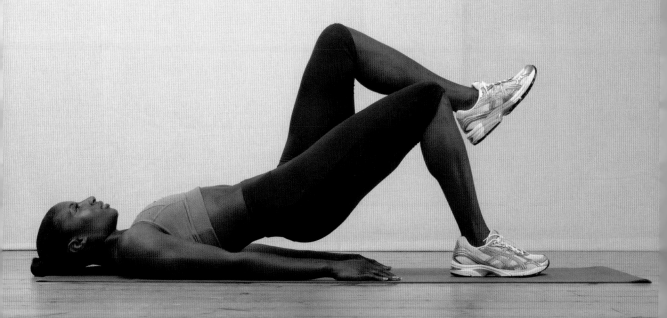

Knee Rocks

For the Front and Deep muscles

1   Lie on your back, knees bent and arms out to the sides, palms flat on the floor.

2   Put your feet in the air, with your knees slightly bent.

3   Lower your feet slowly towards the floor as far as you can.

4   Raise your feet back towards the ceiling until your hips lift off the floor.

Repeat.

> TRAINING TIP
> **Tilt your pelvis towards the ceiling, and maintain the tilt throughout the exercise.**

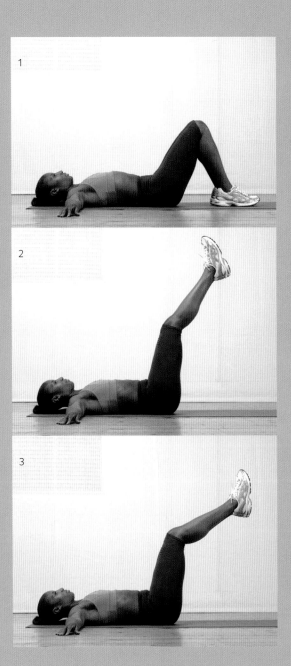

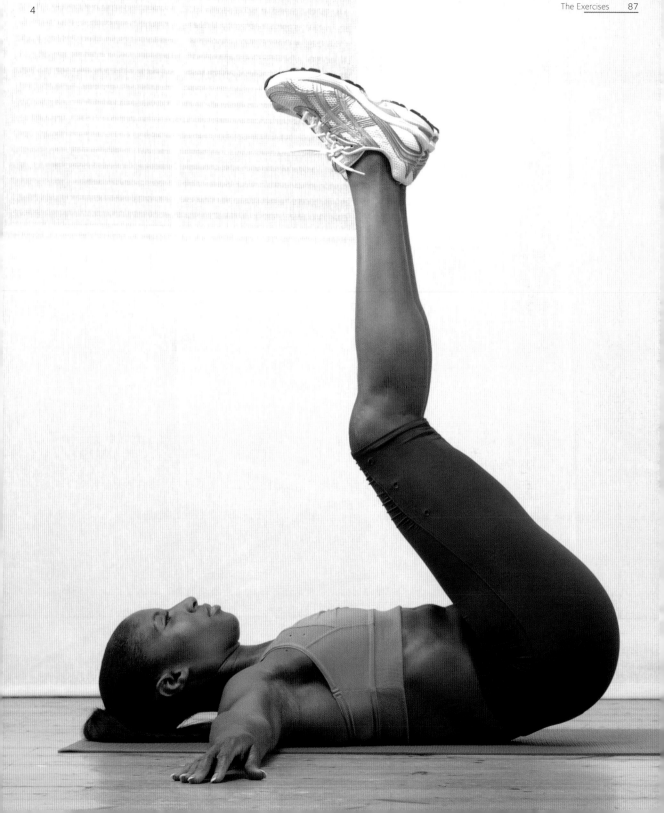

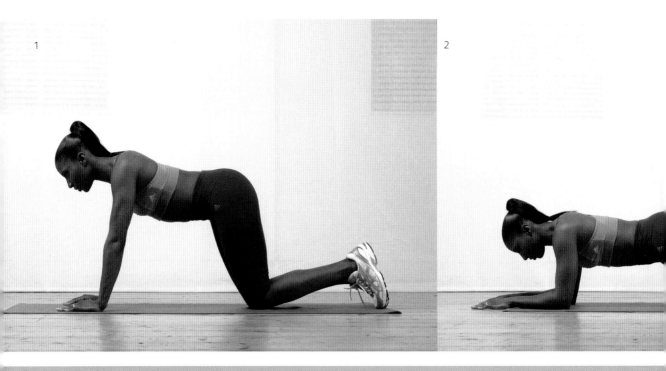

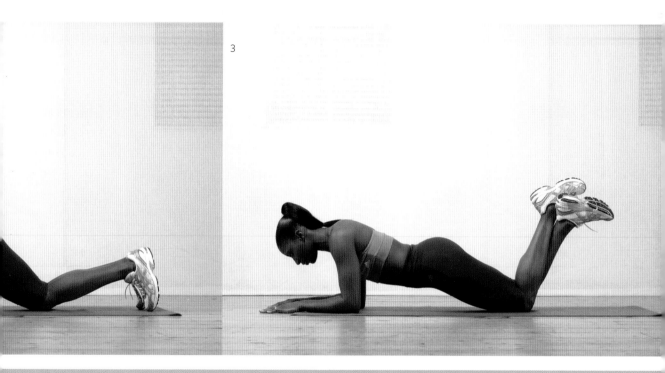

3

Plank

For the Front, Side and Deep muscles

1   Start on all fours with knees together.

2   Drop to your elbows so that you are resting on your elbows and knees, keeping your back flat and tummy tucked in.

3   Lift your feet into the air at about forty-five degrees, ankles crossed. Looking down, keep your torso still and your head straight in alignment with your tailbone. Keep your tummy and buttocks tightened, and hold this position.

Advanced Plank

For the Front, Side and Deep muscles

1   Start on all fours with your knees together.

2   Drop to your elbows so that you are resting on your elbows and knees, keeping your back flat and tummy tucked in.

3   Straighten both legs, taking your weight on your elbows and toes. Keep your body straight and parallel to the floor and your tummy and buttocks tightened, and hold.

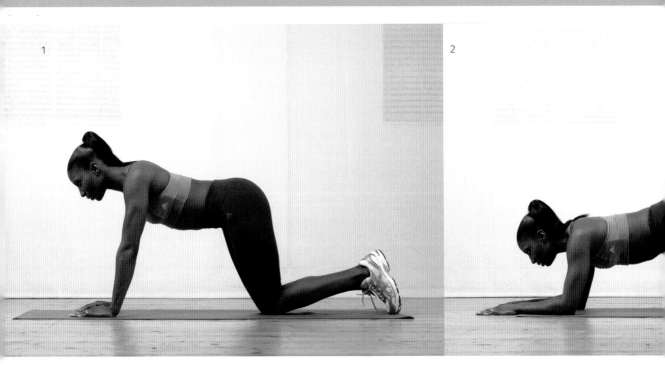

1

2

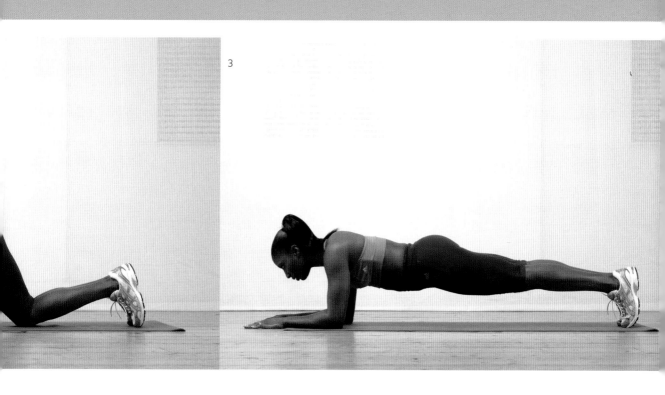

3

1

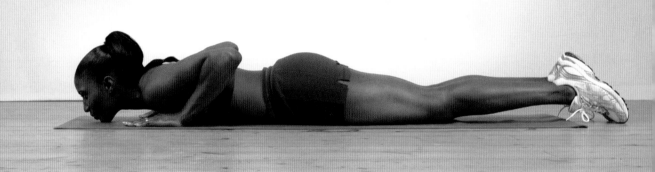

Simple Back Raise

For the Back muscles

1   Lie face down, with your chin on the floor. Bend your
    arms, palms flat to the floor shoulder-width apart.

2   Push up through your hands until your arms are
    straight, pause for a second, then lower to the floor.

    Repeat.

2

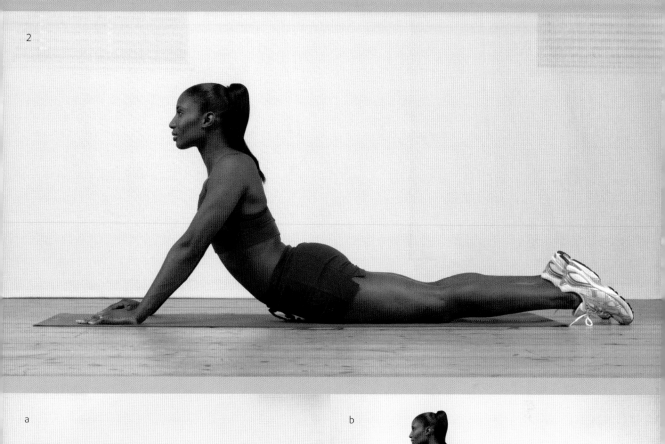

a

b

NOTE

If you have poor range of movement in your back, you can start with your hands level with your head and try to get your arms as straight as possible (figures a & b), then lower to the floor and repeat.

Intermediate Back Raise

For the Back muscles and Glutes

1   Lie face down, your arms straight in front of you
    and your legs straight behind.

2   Squeeze your buttocks to start the movement,
    then raise your arms and feet simultaneously to
    about 10 cm off the floor. Pause for a second
    and return to the starting position.

    Repeat.

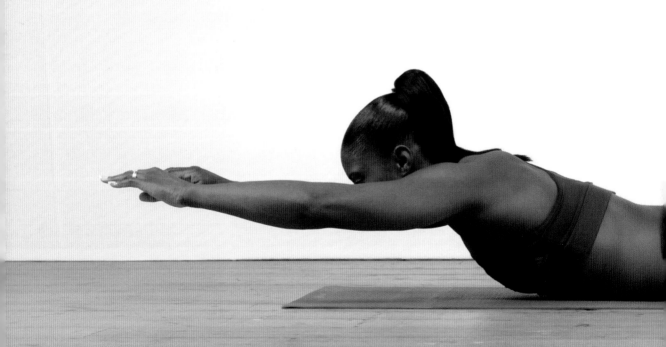

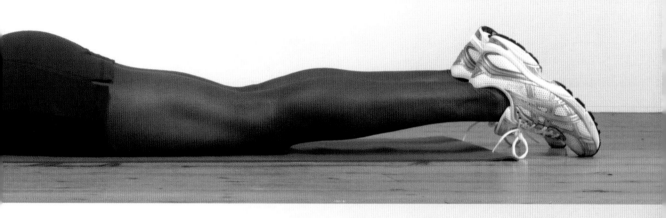

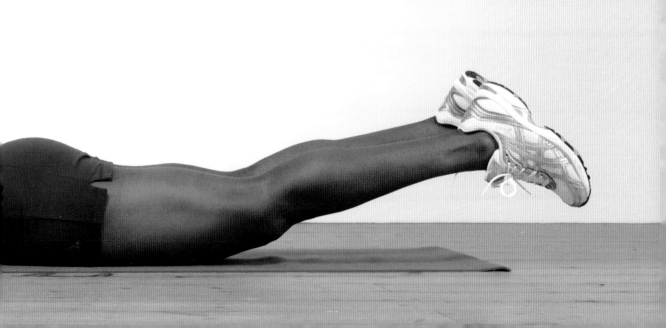

1

Advanced Back Raise

For the Side and Back muscles

1   Lie face down with your forehead touching the floor,
    your hands gently clasped behind your head and
    elbows on the floor, legs straight behind you.

2   Keep looking down as you raise your forehead and
    elbows off the floor.

3   Touch the floor with your right elbow.

4   Touch the floor with your left elbow.

    Return to the centre position, lower your forehead
    and elbows to the floor and repeat.

TRAINING TIP
Keeping your buttocks tight in the movement will
help minimise pressure on your back.

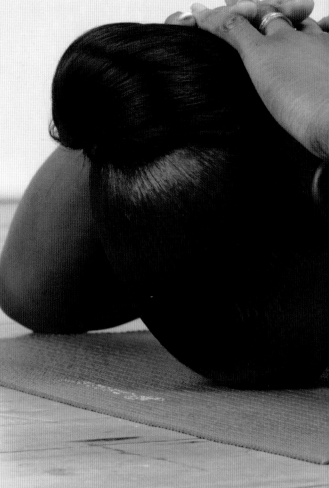

2

3

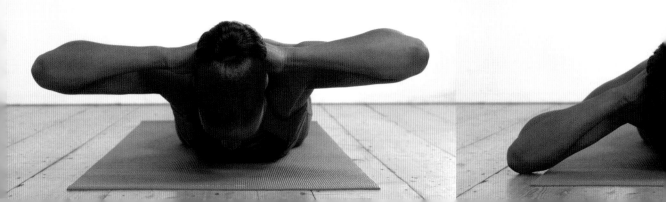

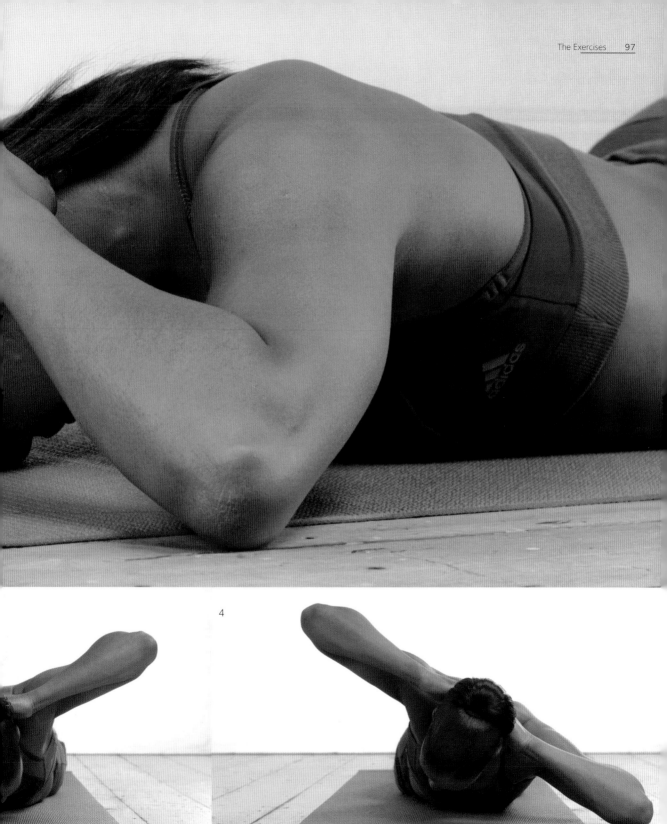

4

Swimming

For the Side, Back, Glutes and Shoulder muscles

1   Lie face down, with your forehead on the floor, arms stretched in front of you, legs out behind.

2   Tightening your buttocks, raise your left leg and right arm simultaneously 10 cm off the floor.

3   As you lower your left leg and right arm, simultaneously raise your right leg and left arm

Repeat, just as if you were paddling, keeping arms and legs straight and avoiding contact with the floor.

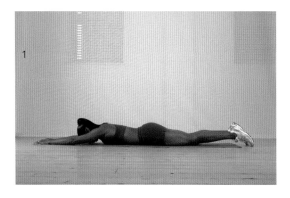

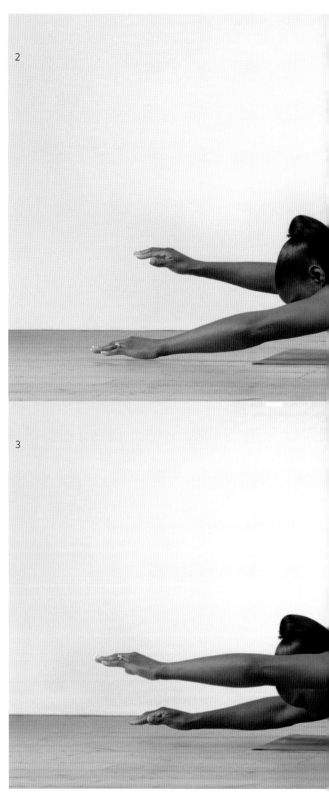

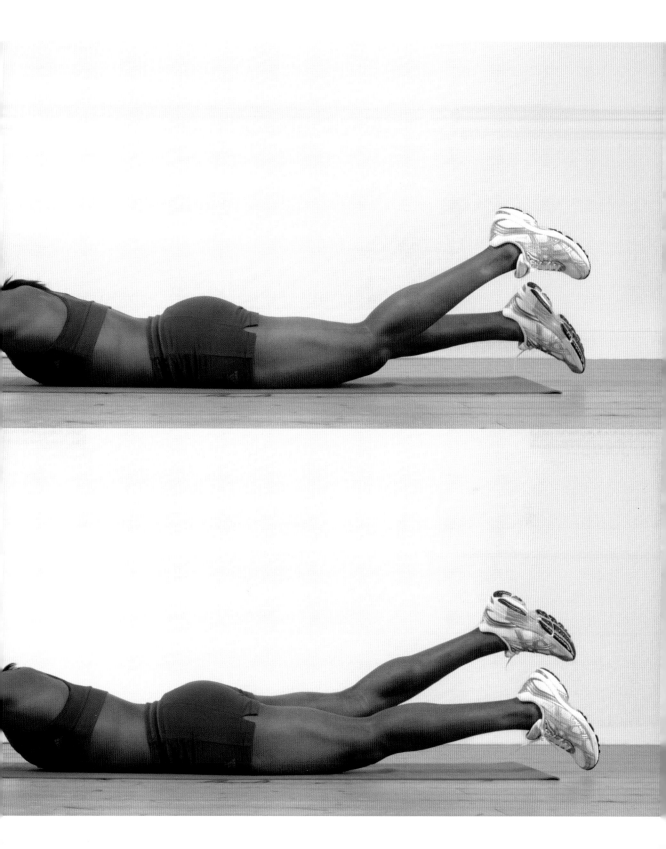

Cool Down

For the cool down you're going to do a gentle form of stretching, and concentrate on slow, deep breathing. Stretching will relieve any muscle soreness produced by the exercises and deep breathing will help to re-energise the system in a way similar to yoga.

At the end of the cool down your body temperature and heart rate will have returned to normal, and your muscles should feel relaxed. I have found that the cooling down period is a good opportunity to make the transition in your mind from exercising to planning the things you need to do during the rest or the day or evening.

You may want to put on a t-shirt before you cool down as your body temperature will be dropping and you could feel a little chilly by the end.

All the exercises should be done in your own time and with control. Take long deep breaths in through the nose and slowly out through the mouth, this will help lower your heart rate and relax you.

To start, lie still for a few moments until you are feeling nice and relaxed in your face, neck, arms, legs and back.

To loosen your back

1   Lie on your back, arms by your sides, knees bent
    and feet flat on the floor.

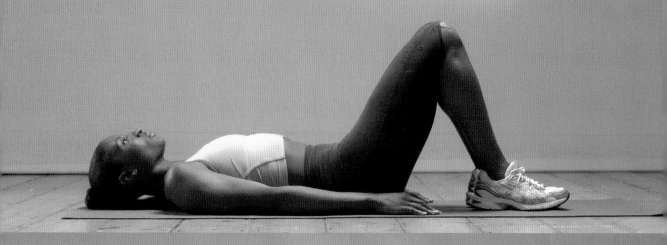

2   Slowly draw up your knees towards your chest,
    hold for 5 seconds and release, returning your
    feet to the floor.

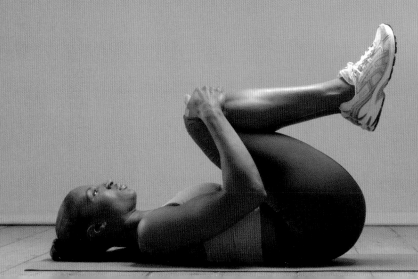

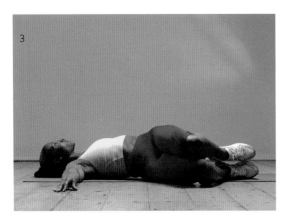

To stretch your sides and lower back

Lie on your back, arms out to the sides, knees bent and feet flat on the floor.

3 Keeping your shoulders flat and your head straight, lower both knees to the right side and hold for 5 seconds.

Raise the knees back to the centre, then lower them to the left side and hold for 5 seconds.

To stretch your abs (1)

Lie face down, with your chin on the floor. Bend your arms, with palms flat to the floor shoulder width apart.

4 Push up through your hands until your arms are straight, hold for 3 seconds, go back down and relax, go up again, hold for 3 seconds and back down again.

To stretch your sides

Sit on your right buttock, knees together and bent, and lower your upper body onto your forearm. Make sure your body is straight, with your tummy tucked in.

5 Extend your left arm above your head, reaching out beyond it, and hold for between 5 and 10 seconds. Repeat on the other side.

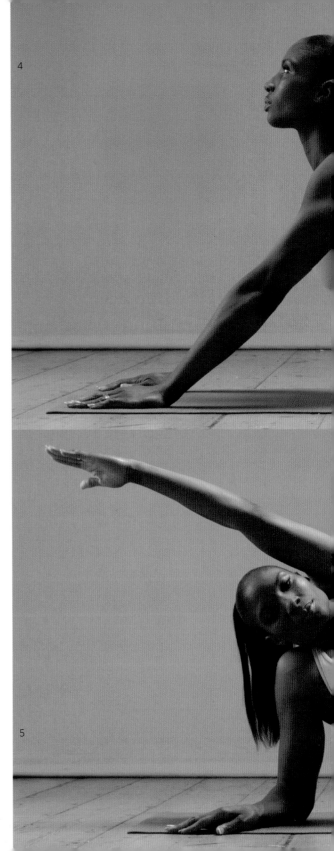

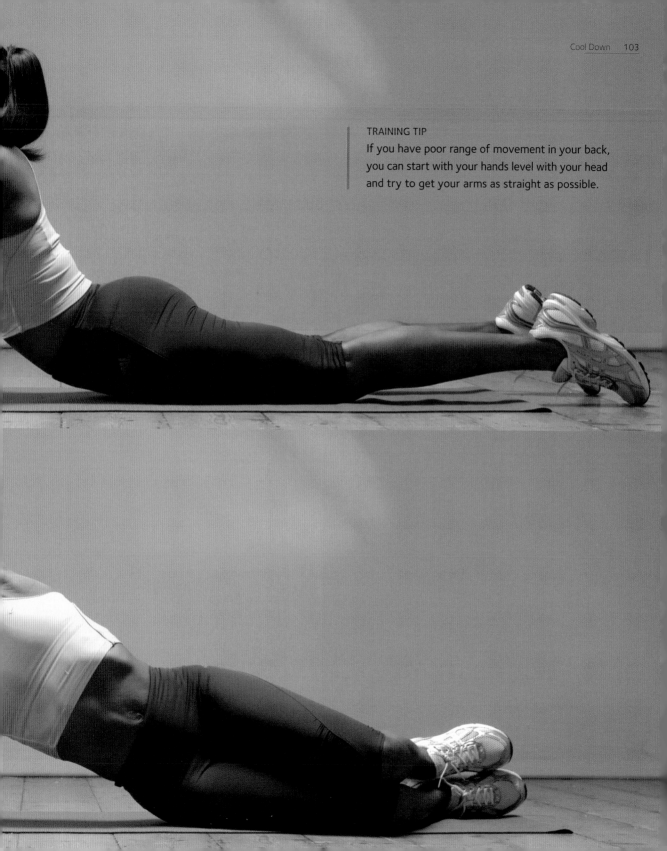

TRAINING TIP
If you have poor range of movement in your back,
you can start with your hands level with your head
and try to get your arms as straight as possible.

To stretch your abs (2)

6   Lie on your back, arms and legs stretched out and
     try to reach as far as possible with your fingers to
     stretch your abs. Hold for 10 seconds.

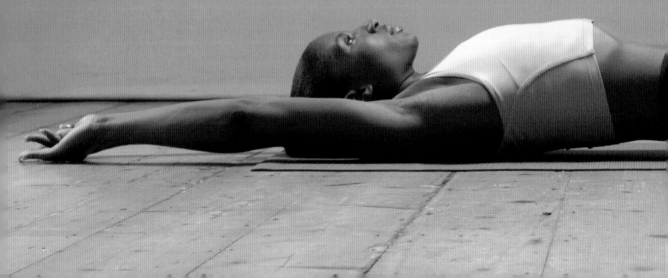

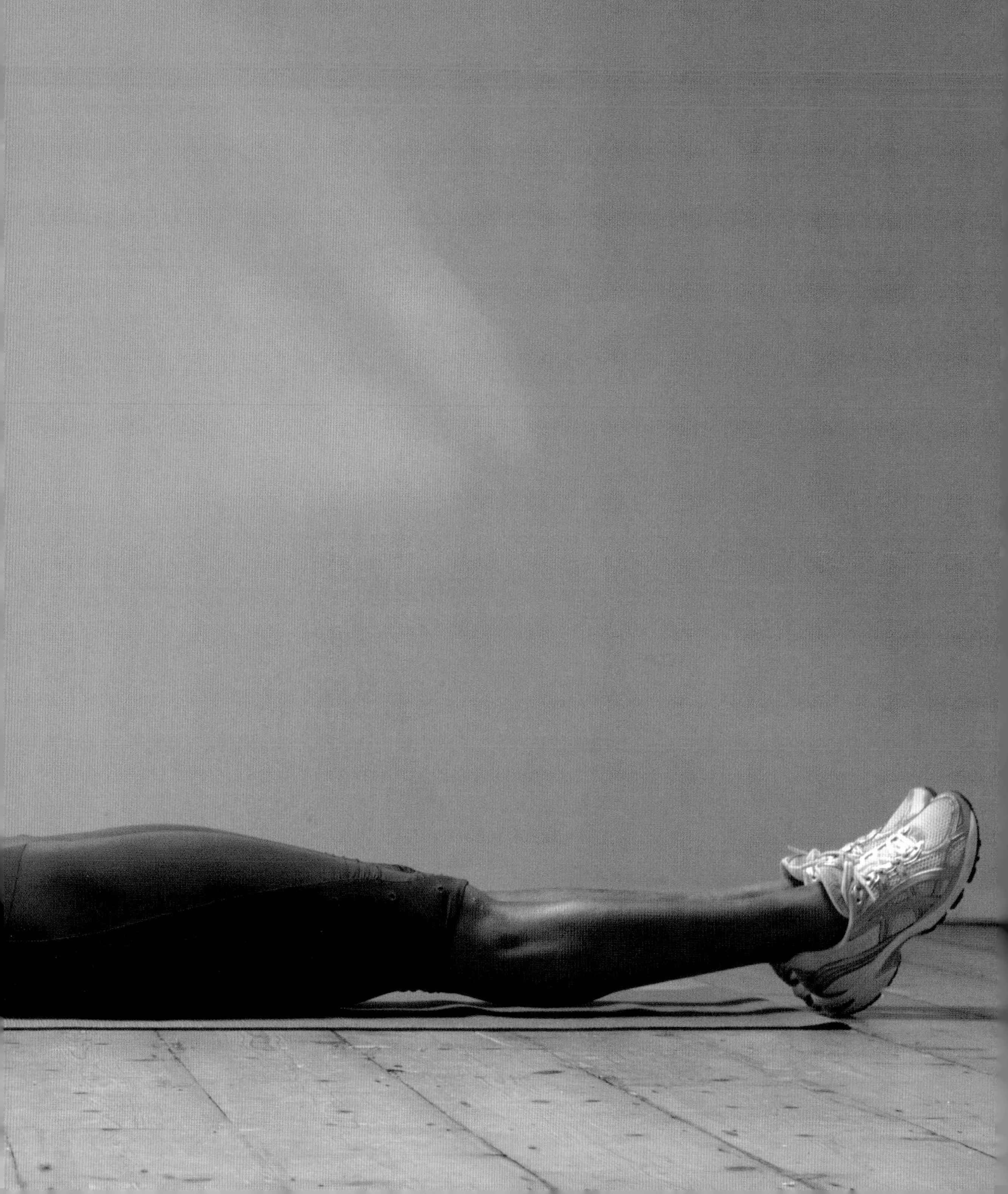

The Programmes

Congratulations for getting to this stage, you have successfully gone through the exercises three or four times and you are ready to take on the programmes.

The exercises have been grouped according to the level of difficulty but moving from beginner through to advanced should be a smooth and easy transition if you commit to doing the programmes regularly.

Each programme will start with a dynamic warm up, a stretching routine and then the exercises themselves followed by a cool down

It is important for you to understand that I have only given you a structured starting point. From there you can develop your workouts.

The number of times that you perform each exercise (reps) can be increased or your recovery times decreased when you get fitter and more confident. If you feel that you want to lengthen your overall workout time, try doing two dynamic warm up exercises instead of one – it will be up to you, but make these changes small and one at a time.

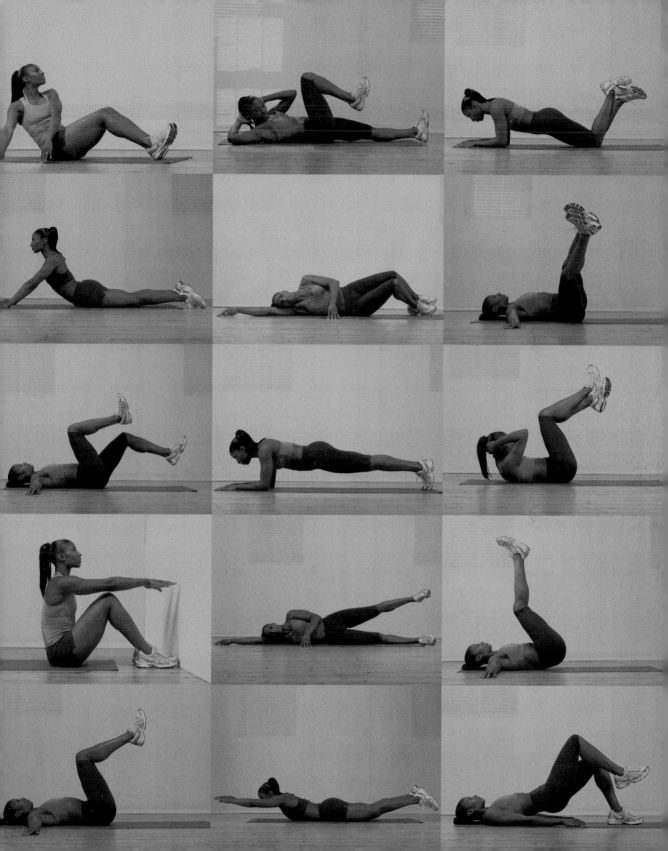

Beginner's Programme 2-3 times a week
Warm up Stretches Exercises Cool down

Dymanic Warm Up
See pages 26-31

Jogging on the spot
See page 28

Skipping
See page 29

Choose ONE of the following:

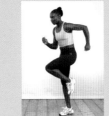

10 secs easy;
10 secs fast;
30 secs rest;
x4

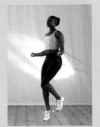

x20 skips;
30 secs rest;
x4

Side Lunges
See page 30
20 secs on; 20 secs rest; x4

Stretches
See pages 32-39

Knee Lifts
See page 42
x10 reps

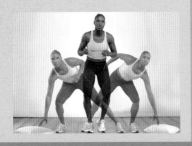

Repeat each stretch 2 or 3 times, depending on how you feel

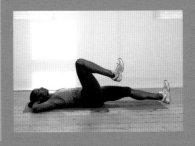

Bent Knee Wipers
See page 48
x10 reps

Open/Close Knees
See page 52
x10 reps

Upper Trunk Rotations
See page 56
x10 reps each side

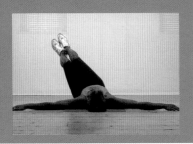

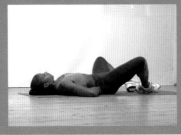

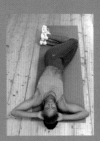

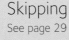

Leg Rotations
See page 58
x10 reps each side

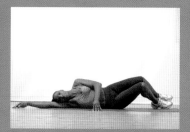

Straight Leg Lifts
See page 60
x10 reps each side

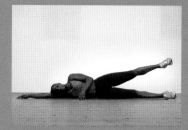

Seated Floor Touches
See page 64
x10 reps

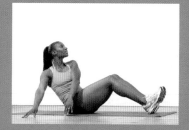

Seated Heal Touches
See page 70
x10 reps each side

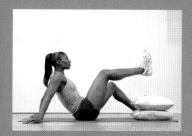

Kneeling Side Bends
See page 74
x10 reps each side

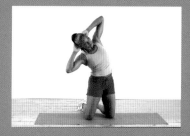

Seated Wall Touches
See page 80
x10 reps

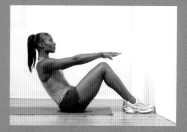

Knee Rocks
See page 86
x10 reps

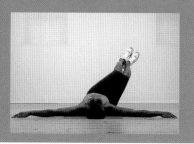

Simple Back Raise
See page 92
x10 reps

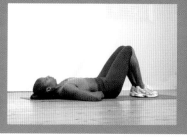

Cool Down
See pages 100–105

Slowly repeat each stretch
2 or 3 times, depending
on how you feel

Intermediate Programme 2-3 times a week

Warm up Stretches Exercises Cool down

Dymanic Warm Up
See pages 26-31

Jogging on the Spot
See page 28

Skipping
See page 29

Choose ONE of the following:

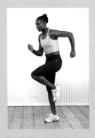

20 secs easy;
10 secs fast;
20 secs easy;
10 secs fast;
30 secs rest;
x3-4

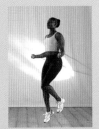

x40 skips;
60 secs rest;
x3

Side Lunges
See page 30
30 secs on; 30 secs rest; x4

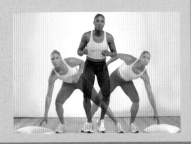

Stretches
See pages 32-39

Repeat each stretch 2 or 3 times,
depending on how you feel

Advanced Knee Lifts
See page 44
x10 reps

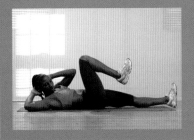

Bicycle
See page 46
x10 reps

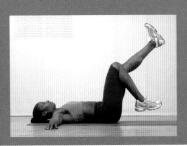

Bent Knee Wipers
See page 48
x10 reps

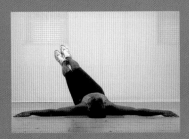

Advanced Open/Close
Knees See page 54
x10 reps

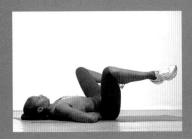

Upper Trunk Rotations
See page 56
x10 reps each side

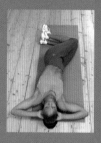

Advanced Straight Leg Lifts See page 62
x10 reps each side

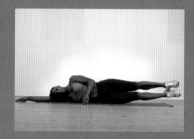

Intermediate Floor Touches See page 66
x10 reps

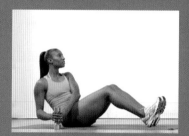

Seated Heel Touches
See page 70
x10 reps each side

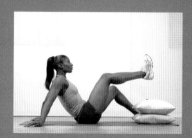

Intermediate Side Bends
See page 76
x10 reps

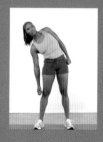

Simple Crunches
See page 82
x10 reps

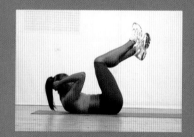

Plank
See page 88
Hold for 30 secs

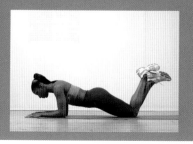

Intermediate Back Raise See page 94
x10 reps

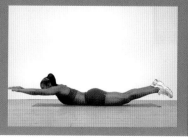

Cool Down
See pages 100-105

Slowly repeat each stretch
2 or 3 times, depending
on how you feel

Advanced Programme 2-3 times a week
Warm up Stretches Exercises Cool down

Dymanic warm up
See pages 26-31

Jogging on the spot
See page 28

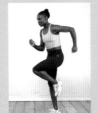

10 secs easy;
10 secs fast;
30 secs rest;
x4

Skipping
See page 29

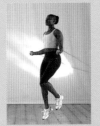

x20 skips;
30 secs rest;
x4

Choose ONE of the following:

Side lunges
See page 30
20 secs on; 20 secs rest; x4

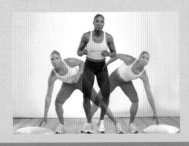

Stretches
See pages 32-39

Repeat each stretch 2 or 3 times, depending on how you feel

Advanced Knee Lifts
See page 44
x10 reps

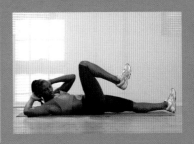

Bicycle
See page 46
x10 reps

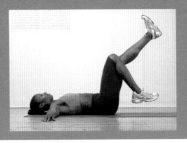

Straight Leg Wipers
See page 50
x10 reps

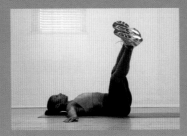

Advanced Back Raise
See page 96
x 5 reps

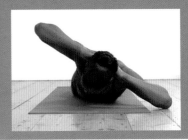

Advanced Open/Close Knees See page 54
x10 reps

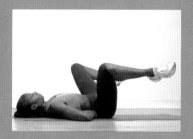

Advanced Straight Leg Lifts See page 62
x10 reps each side

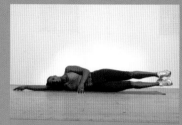

Advanced Floor Touches See page 68
x10 reps

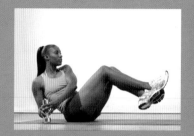

Advanced Heel Touches
See page 72
x10 reps

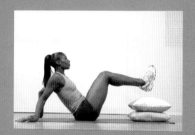

Swimming
See page 98
20 seconds

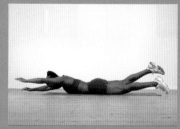

Advanced Side Bends
See page 78
x10 reps

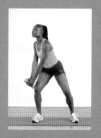

Hip Raise with Knee Lift See page 84
x10 reps

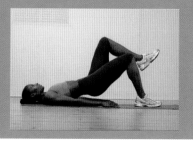

Advanced Plank
See page 90
Hold for 30 secs

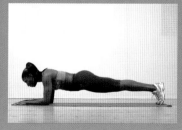

Cool Down
See pages 100-105

Slowly repeat each stretch
2 or 3 times, depending
on how you feel

Staying With It

'After a few weeks on the programmes, the rewards of staying with it will be there for you to see with your own eyes because you'll be looking good. Hopefully this will be all the encouragement you need.'

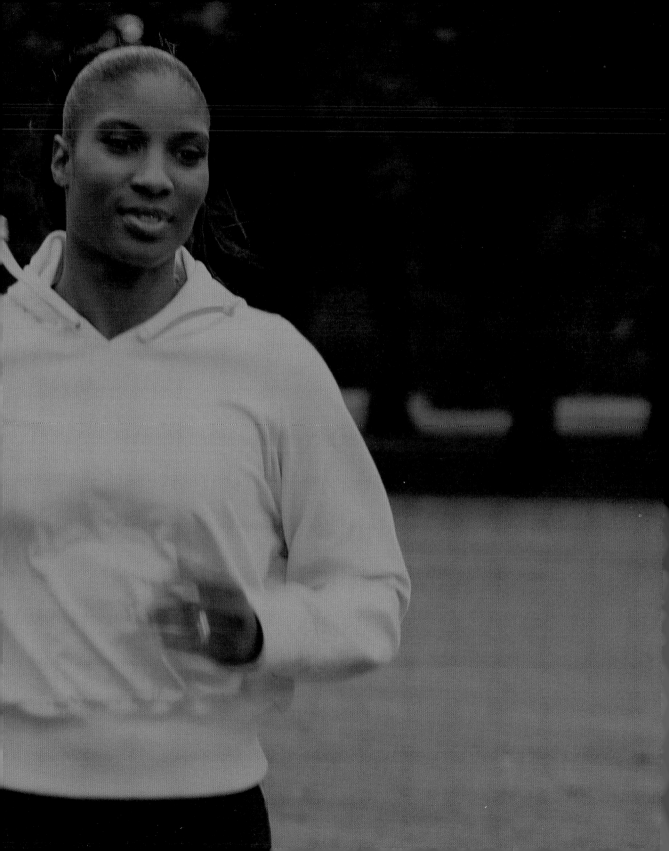

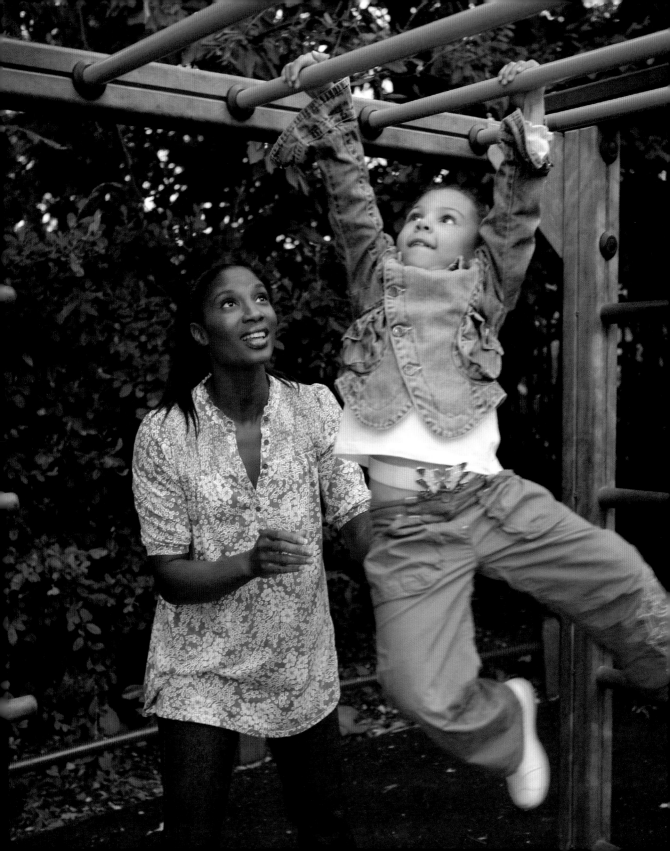

Keeping going, keep moving on

Congratulations, you're exercising! You've made room for exercise in your lifestyle and you'll soon see the benefits. You're only four to six weeks away from becoming fitter and stronger and you're well on the way to getting the flat tummy you want.

Exercising will get easier as you progress, so the programmes are designed to keep you engaged and hopefully if you are managing to do them two or three times a week you'll be able to move from beginner through intermediate to advanced level comfortably. If you've been finding it hard to keep going, get a friend involved: a mutual appointment to exercise can be all the encouragement you need.

If you have never kept a diary before you may find this a useful tool. I kept a training diary for over fifteen years, recording my training and competition results, my eating patterns, my mood and general wellbeing. Keeping a diary is a great way of monitoring your progress and will give you the opportunity to discover patterns in your week that you may not have noticed otherwise.

After a few weeks, the rewards of staying with it will be there for you to see with your own eyes because you'll be looking good. Hopefully this will be all the encouragement you need. I would like to think that your confidence is growing and maybe you are considering branching out and trying something a little more adventurous.

Maybe you could introduce other forms of exercising that suit you, like joining a local gym that offers a wide range of fitness classes. You might try adding some prolonged cardiovascular exercise such as jogging, cycling, or swimming. These are general forms of conditioning and can go a long way towards controlling your overall weight. They are complete body workouts and good for the heart and lungs.

You could even do something totally different like indoor rock climbing or rowing. If you have children and they are old enough, take them with you, make exercising fun: it doesn't have to be a chore.

Food for Thought

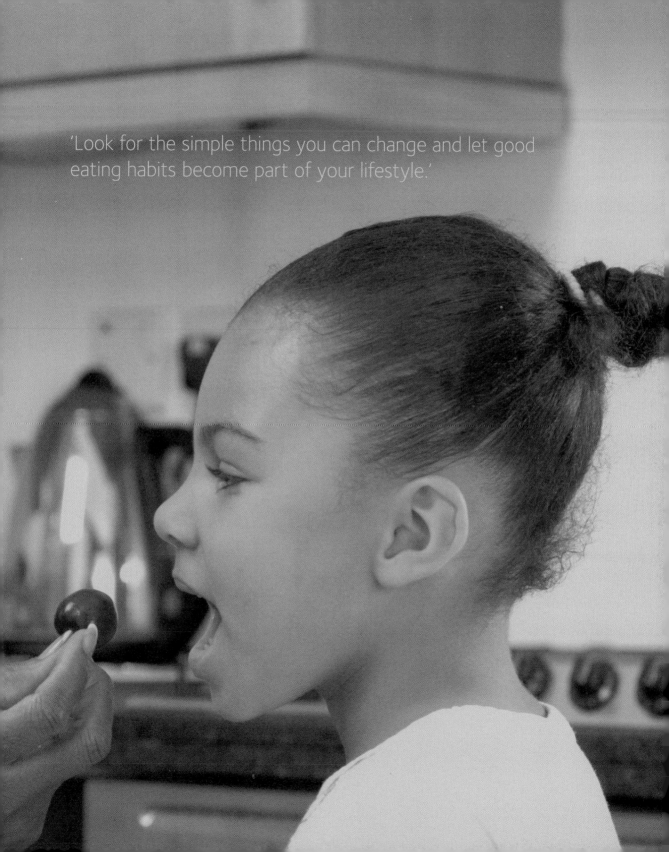

'Look for the simple things you can change and let good eating habits become part of your lifestyle.'

Eating sensibly + exercise = a healthier you

I love to eat, so I have never been fond of books about dieting. You don't need to deny yourself food to stay in shape. You can indulge a healthy appetite simply by exercising regularly and being prepared to improve what you eat.

Frankly, I don't know how I won my first major championship at the Commonwealth Games in 1994 because my lifestyle and eating habits were really bad. I was eating burgers, fish and chips and chicken sandwiches with lashings of mayonnaise. But after 1994, I met a great nutritionist, who steered me in the right direction and opened my eyes to the power of eating the right food.

It took me a year to really adjust my eating habits, but what a difference fuelling myself correctly made. I went from not having enough energy to train twice a day to being able to sustain and recover from double sessions every day. Because I was getting all the goodness I needed through my food, when I trained I was no longer breaking down valuable muscle tissue, enabling me to become fitter and stronger.

I no longer need the same rigidity as I did back then, but my athlete's understanding of how to eat still helps me enjoy food without piling on the pounds.

I've proposed throughout the book that having goals is essential. This is as true about what you eat as it is about how you exercise. Look for the simple changes you can make straight away and let good eating habits become part of your lifestyle.

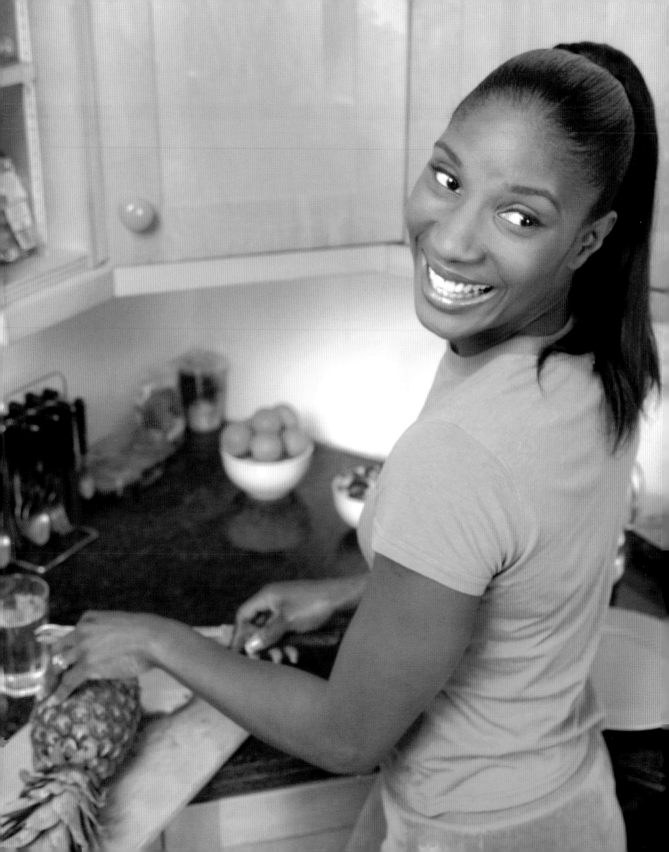

Here are some suggestions for simple changes that will help give you more energy for work, exercise and life.

· Changing your eating habits is not easy, so keep it simple to start with. For example, swapping refined sugar for brown sugar or changing your bread from white to brown are easy things you can achieve.

· Don't stint on breakfast. It's the most important meal because it sets you up for the rest of the day, whether a full day at work or at home with the kids.

· Try some warm water and lemon juice in the morning. It's a simple but effective way to cleanse your system.

· Fit your eating pattern to your workout time, making sure you've got good food in your system to give you much more energy to exercise.

· Unless you have the time and really love cooking, try to make lunch simple, manageable and as healthy as possible. And if you're eating sandwiches because that's all you fancy, try to have pitta bread or make an open sandwich, using one slice of bread instead of two.

· Using small dinner plates really does work!

· You can graze a bit through the day. I find grazing beneficial when I'm really busy. It helps to control the blood sugar levels, so you don't have the urge for something sweet to get that instant fix. Unsalted nuts, dried and fresh fruit are good for this.

- Between lunch and the evening meal is the longest part of the day without food for most people, and between four and five in the afternoon you're probably at your hungriest with a lot still to do before you can tuck into a proper meal, so it's good to have healthy snack foods to hand.

- Try not to drink too much coffee, black tea and fizzy drinks all day.

- Preparation is king: help yourself by not putting the things you know you need to cut down on into your shopping trolley. In fact avoid those aisles completely. Try to buy your chosen snack food in advance for the week.

- If you must treat yourself, do it at the weekends, you are after all only human.

- In some instances you might want to look at the type of food you're eating, for example too much stodgy food makes you feel lethargic.

- Water is your friend so drink it. I'm not sure why, but I can never seem to drink enough water if I drink it from a glass, so I tend to re-fill bottles of water so I can measure how much I'm drinking. Aiming for two litres is about right.

- You may find that asking for a little help from your friends and your partner will help to keep you from temptation.

Exercise and You

'Exercising will probably feel difficult at first, but after
a few attempts, the body will get used to working out.
After 20 or so sessions, it will expect it!'

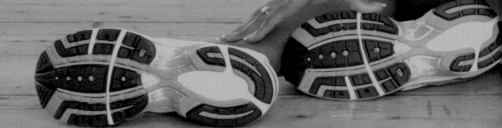

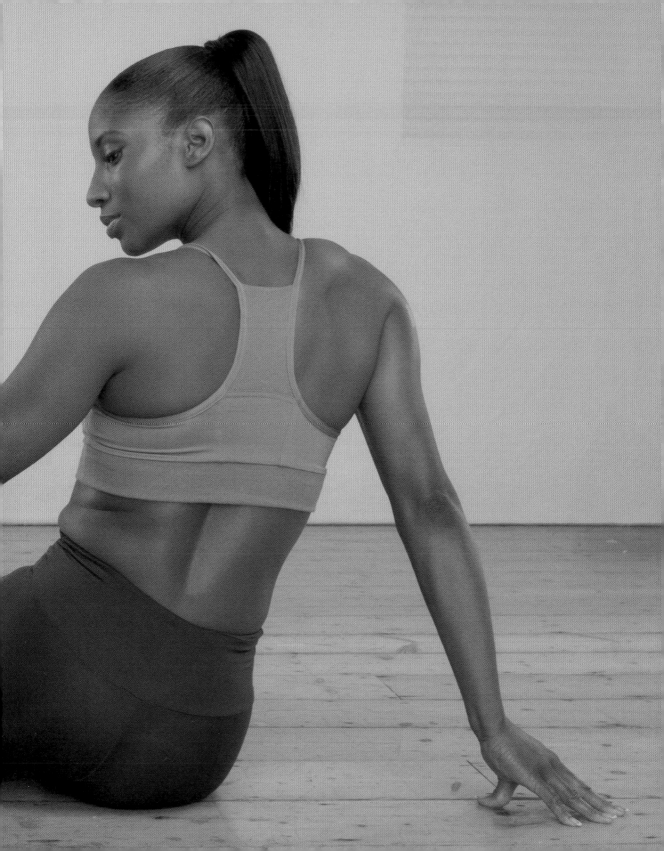

Exercise and you

The exercises in **The Flat Tummy Book** have mostly been about getting strong abs and a beautiful flat tummy but they will benefit you in other ways too.

- Exercising will probably feel difficult at first, but after a few attempts, the body will get used to working out. After 20 or so sessions, it will expect it!

- Working out expands your sense of well-being because the production of endorphins, chemicals released naturally by the brain, increases after exercise: like anything in life, you have to do the hard bit before you get the good bit. Once you've had that endorphin kick, you'll think, 'oh that's nice' and want to do it again.

- Exercising gets the best out of the heart and lungs because we're actually extending their capacity to cope with everyday things like running for the bus, climbing a load of stairs, or walking down those long airport terminals.

- The metabolism is the vital process that converts food into energy and this slows down naturally with age. Exercise can speed up the process and help make it easier to burn the calories.

- I'd think about exercising sooner rather than later because as time goes on it gets harder to keep your body in shape and the things you've taken for granted become more difficult to maintain: skin and muscles give up their elasticity and recovery from injury takes longer.

- Exercise is a valuable aid through the menopause, when your body needs to be strengthened to deal with its changes.

- If your tummy muscles are not activated, they'll lose their tension. They're almost like armour supporting the skeleton and if they're strong and work in harmony with the back muscles, you'll have great posture and fluidity of movement. In 2004 this core strength gave me the advantage over the other female celebrity dancers of Strictly Come Dancing and allowed me to maintain a very good 'ballroom hold'.

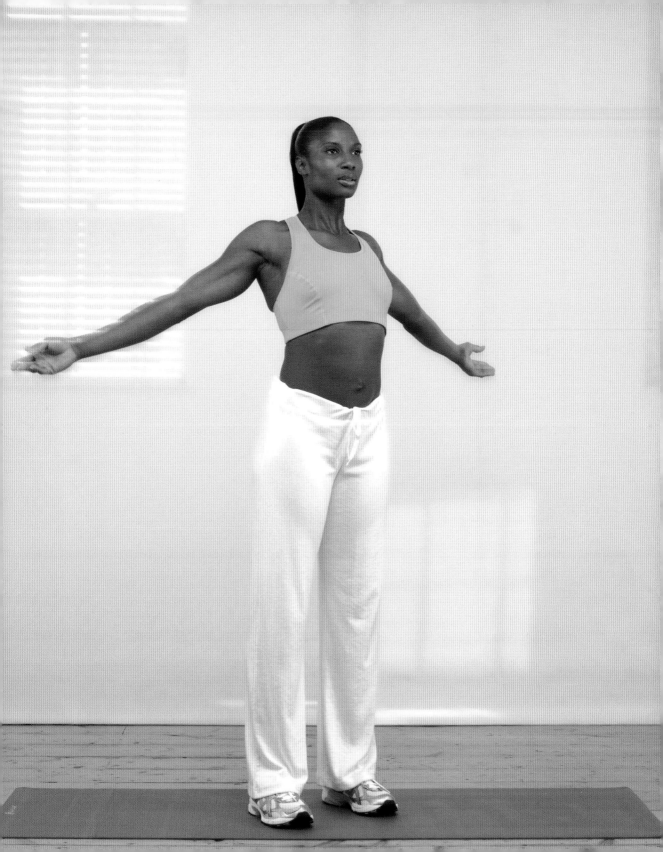

Credits

Quercus
21 Bloomsbury Square
London, WC1A 2NS

First published in 2008

A catalogue record for this book is available from the British Library.
ISBN: 978-1-905204-50-2

Book design: Grade Design Consultants, London
Photography: Mike Prior
Hair and make-up: Andrew Savage
Editorial: Philippa Brewster

Printed and bound in Italy